A GRAND
SLAM
LIFE

A Physician Gets COVID, Finds His Way,
and Works to Transform a Texas Community

Milton Haber, M.D. with Beth Herman

authorHOUSE®

AuthorHouse™
1663 Liberty Drive
Bloomington, IN 47403
www.authorhouse.com
Phone: 833-262-8899

Published by AuthorHouse 06/24/2021

ISBN: 978-1-6655-2878-8 (sc)
ISBN: 978-1-6655-2876-4 (hc)
ISBN: 978-1-6655-2877-1 (e)

Library of Congress Control Number: 2021911846

Print information available on the last page.

Photo cover by Jose "Joe" Sillas.

This book is printed on acid-free paper.

Contents

Dedication vii

Prologue...ix

Chapter 1   In the Beginning...1

Chapter 2   In the Clearing 13

Chapter 3   In the Thick of It...23

Chapter 4   In the Process 33

Chapter 5   In the ACTS 47

Chapter 6   In the Zone..57

Chapter 7   In the Lab...73

Chapter 8   In the Light 83

Chapter 9   In a Post-COVID World 93

Acknowledgments 105

About the Author 107

Dedication

This book is dedicated to the future of clinical trials
and its role in making the world a better place.

Prologue

I've often wondered why people write a book. Is it a passion they have? A burning desire to right some wrong? Valuable lessons that should be shared? Is there an inspiring story that needs to be told? Perhaps it's a simple, earnest attempt to plant the seeds of change. For me, it was all of the above. The catalyst, however, was getting the coronavirus myself. As a practicing internist in Laredo, Texas, and Founding Owner and President of Laguna Clinical Research Associates, LLC—a medical research company helping execute the Moderna COVID-19 vaccine trials, experiencing the virus gave me insights I'd never have had on the outside looking in. But that's only part of the story.

Newly approved for Emergency Use Authorization (EUA), when the approved vaccine arrived in Laredo, I'd just come through a debilitating few weeks of fevers, fatigue, and a crushing weakness that caused me to fall and strike my chest and abdomen on an iron bedpost. I cut myself up and broke my third, fourth, and seventh ribs. I was hospitalized. Turns out I had pneumonia and there were other issues I will talk about later in the book.

I returned to work just as twenty-five hundred cars queued up for five hundred doses of the vaccine. I was equal parts elated and heartbroken. Help for my community was finally here and people had really gotten the message my research company had tried so hard to convey amid controversy about the readiness of the vaccine: that people needed to trust science. We were doing something productive and people turned out, yet with this shortage we were falling shy of our goal.

Barely recovered and not at my strongest, nevertheless all day I moved from car to car, thanking people and reassuring the ones turned away that one way or another, if they stayed committed and stayed the course, life would surely change for them. I cared and would never give up.

Laredo is an underserved community. The clinical trials my research company got to administer were in themselves a gift because historically, less than 1 percent of Latino and Black populations participate in clinical trials. When Moderna selected Laguna from a large number of interested venues, I was quite proactive, going on TV and social media to promote the importance of the study to the community and how fortunate Laredo was to have been selected to participate. Despite the politics of it all, you'll see me say a number of times throughout the book that we need to trust science. It helped when Dr. Anthony Fauci, Director of the National Institute of Allergy and Infectious Diseases, put pressure on Moderna to increase its enrollment, which opened the door to expanded recruitment efforts trickling down to us in Laredo. It was an unprecedented opportunity here to change people's lives, and for me to serve my community in the process.

But how and why did I get involved in clinical trials to begin with, and why does my story matter?

Since 1987, my internal medicine practice has grown from a first day grand total of thirteen patients to twelve thousand. I was proud of the hard work that went into building this practice because again, so much of my community is marginalized. I was born and raised in a hard-working Laredo family, and in addition to my Hippocratic Oath, if my patients were hungry there was no way I wasn't going to feed them. If they lacked funds to pay the landlord, I was going to help them see to that too. You've heard of doctors who practice holistic medicine, treating not just the symptoms of the disease but the whole patient. Well, you might say—and all too often to my accountant's dismay—that I practice holistic everything. I'm just one person, not a foundation or institution, but I've always tried to go beyond treating illness into treating humanity. It's one thing to get medication but if you can't keep the lights on to see well enough to see the label, what's the point? I also hoped to be an example for my children and others who may be paying attention, to help them understand that as human beings we are not separate. Pain, lack, and suffering are universal conditions. Each of us doing what we can to alleviate it—whatever form that takes—should also be a universal condition. So I've spent three decades trying. Yet, over time, somehow I felt what I was doing on my own wasn't enough. There were times I felt as though I was just wallowing around in the water.

In 2019, in tandem with Veronica Procasky, a gifted and visionary attorney and nurse who would later become my company's CEO (more about our propitious meeting later in the book), we started Laguna Clinical Research Associates, LLC. As a medical research company, Laguna qualifies to conduct clinical trials that will ultimately benefit hundreds of thousands of people—clearly more than the number of patients I got to help from time to time.

I have always believed the direction of our lives is decided long before we live them in a kind of life script. Our lives are predestined. If we deviate from the script, life gets off track and we're flailing, and if we're honest with ourselves we know it. We generally follow the script, though, and for me, years later, I felt a calling to be part of something bigger, which turned out to be research and clinical trials.

As the Fates would have it, soon after Laguna Research was established, COVID-19 hit. When we were sanctioned to help execute the Moderna vaccine trials, I had an emotional reaction. I knew the results of our research would be immediate. People beyond the trial participants would get help—our country needed help—and not years down the road as happens with most clinical trials. The average timetable in terms of vaccine development is five to ten years. The coronavirus vaccine was developed and implemented in about seven months.

Though we are on the right path, I have deep concerns about the fallout from the coronavirus. At this time, inevitably, the number and variations of comorbidities—the ways in which COVID-19 may affect our hearts, gastrointestinal, nervous, and reproductive systems, brain function, etc.—are both incalculable and incomprehensible. The medical landscape, political or otherwise, will undergo radical change. Its economic impact is something of which we can't yet fully conceive. Every human being on this earth will be impacted by the coronavirus for years to come. Our ability to anticipate, project, pivot, and effectively meet the challenges, as well as our willingness to extend ourselves in whatever ways we can to help others, will be the key to our survival. This will also be the key to our happiness so that each of us can fulfill our purpose on earth.

My profession is rooted in science, traditionally the bastion of dispassionate realists and the like. While I'm a realist myself, I also tend to be more of an optimist, and just maybe a little overboard in my quest to save the world. I want to make sure people know there are thousands of researchers and physicians in this country and elsewhere who do give a damn. They care about outcomes and quality of life. They want to make a difference as much as I do, and though the coronavirus is a bend in the road almost no one could anticipate, we are here to see our patients through it at all costs.

Overall I had a good life growing up but it wasn't without its own set of challenges, the story of which I'll unpack as we move through the book. One thing I learned was the importance of taking care of others.

My mother was born overseas and raised in Mexico before coming to the United States. As a small boy with her en route to visit my grandparents, stopped in a San Luis Potosi train station, I saw a nursing mother propped up in the middle of the floor. She was young but wrinkled beyond belief. She looked beaten down by life, something I'd not seen in my small Texas town, though I'd see more of it as I accompanied my mother across the border more and more. Eventually I came to understand the young woman's life was nothing but extreme hardship. I will never forget the look of utter despair on her face. My mother bought me a Mexican chocolate bar that day and I turned around and gave it to her. Frankly I didn't like Mexican chocolate anyway, so I didn't deserve any kind of *ata' boy* there. But in a kind of baptism by fire, I learned that poverty and pain go hand in hand, deciding that if I could do anything about it—any large or small aspect of it—I simply would.

The fact is I was not a good student prior to medical school, definitely not interested in school at all, and in a million years never thought I was medical school material. This is an unbelievable, against all odds, even humorous story in itself I tell in chapter 2. I can only guess it was written somewhere in my life script that I'd get in, and though I didn't know it at the time, apparently this was the platform I was supposed to use to effect change which I will never stop trying to do.

My story is the journey—snagged, cracked, funny, flawed, and all—I took to get here and continue to take in the wake of a world-changing pandemic. I hope it inspires you to persevere and find your calling as I found mine. We all have a life's purpose and once we discover it, our time on earth becomes vastly different than it was before. Even if my path doesn't immediately motivate you, the message I hope you take away is the significance of taking, without reservation, the life-changing vaccine now being offered. This cannot be overstated. Clearly there are elements of our existence we cannot control. I believe it's up to us, even our responsibility, to embrace the ones we can.

Milton Haber, M.D.
Laredo, Texas
April 15, 2021

1

In the Beginning

"For in every adult there dwells the child that was, and in every child there lies the adult that will be." – John Connolly

We all come from somewhere. Sometimes I think the luckiest of us come from everywhere, or at least have some degree of diversity in our DNA as I do. Maybe it creates a restlessness and complexity in our souls. Poland; Mexico; Syria—that's what I know about myself, though I suspect there are other faraway places.

My mother, Rosa, one of four sisters, was born in a small Polish border town near Russia that the Nazis eventually invaded. Though she left in 1934 when she was just six years old, until the day she died sixty years later she shivered at the memory of the cold, grey, joyless environment in which she lived. You could say she passionately hated it. It wasn't just the oppressive political climate for Jews at the time, though she did recall the prejudice. She felt genuinely suffocated by the ugliness all around her, as though covered by a shroud. Fortunately her father wasn't happy there either. Strongly opposed by her mother, he was adamant about leaving anyway, threatening to take their four daughters and hightail it for America. Her mother eventually relented, a very good thing as much of their family would end up perishing in concentration camps. The saga goes that their ship, en route to the United States, docked first in Veracruz, Mexico. For some reason they got off. Their last name was Marantz, misunderstood by immigration officials, which was often the case, so they became Marac.

In a country teeming with color and celebration, sunlight and warmth, little Rosa Marac recalled feeling alive for the very first time. Though she knew nothing of Christianity and didn't speak a word of Spanish, she and her sisters were enrolled in a Mexican Catholic school, the only school in the area. In time she became completely bilingual in Spanish and of course Yiddish, her native tongue, in which she used to talk to her sisters the whole time I was growing up. In time she learned English but Yiddish was the sisters' code. Along with my sister, brother, and father, I never knew what they were talking about. I guess that was the point.

My Laredo-born father, Maurice, one of six children (a sister died of appendicitis at age thirteen), was born of a resilient, though illiterate, Syrian immigrant father and mother—my paternal grandparents. In the early 1900s, a carpenter by trade, my grandfather and his fourteen-year-old bride immigrated to New York through Ellis Island. Upon arrival, subject as were all foreigners entering this country to strict medical scrutiny by the United States Public Health Service, they were found to have tuberculosis. Subsequently they were held in Ellis Island isolation units on the southern-most wing for two years. When pronounced free of the disease, they paid $1 a week for a Brooklyn hotel, eking out a living as peddlers. Selling whatever they could to survive, the couple eventually peddled their wares all the way down to Texas. At some point in their marriage they divorced, unusual for the times. And from the time I can remember my grandfather lived with us, sleeping in a tiny one-room structure with a shower my father built for him out back. There was no sink so he shaved in a bathroom with a sink inside our house. My father was always ashamed of him, uneducated—I don't think he went past the second grade in Syria—and illiterate at least as far as English was concerned. He didn't want to be anything like this his father though he always took care of him.

In World War II, my father entered the Army Air Force as a navigator and if memory serves me, he became an instructor as well. Returning in one piece to Laredo, he was ready for a wife with the condition that she had to be Jewish. He consulted with his rabbi who promptly sent a telegram to a rabbi in Mexico City where the single Jewish female population was apparently ripe for the picking.

On the appointed day, my father traveled to a Mexico City synagogue to meet a bevy of eligible women. Unfortunately—or fortunately for me, else I'd never have been born— the lineup was unappealing and my temporarily downcast father walked out the door. As I remember it being told, he literally bumped into Rosa, the woman who would become my mother, who worked at the bank next door. To heighten the drama and if you believe as I do in the life script of their meeting, it turns out my mother had not taken her usual route back to the bank, veering from the course. Had she not done that, today you'd not be reading this book because I'd not be here to write it. There's a saying in the Jewish religion: *bashert*, meaning destiny, especially in regard to a soulmate. My father was utterly struck by this beautiful woman who'd crossed his path at exactly the right minute, and who at the time didn't speak a word of English. She was also dating someone considered to be Mexico's version of Walter Cronkite. My parents married three months later on April 18, 1948, my father bringing his new bride home to Laredo.

For the first three years of my big sister Brenda's life, my mother didn't speak a word of English. By the time I was born and in my first years, it was about a seventy/thirty Spanish-English split. You'd think as a result I'd be entirely bilingual but I'm not, though my Latino patients understand my earnest attempts to explain things—or pretend to because they pity me. At least they don't laugh. When my brother Charlie was born two years later, mom was increasingly better at English and as the years passed, when we were in college, she excelled enough to study for her master's degree in art, going to work for the first time, teaching art at the college level.

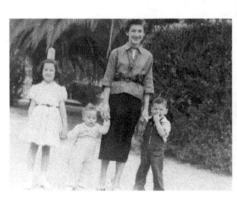
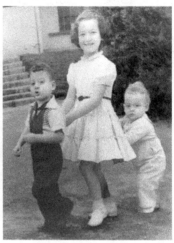

Left: My mother with my sister Brenda, my brother Charlie, and me.
Right: Me, my sister Brenda, and my brother Charlie having fun.

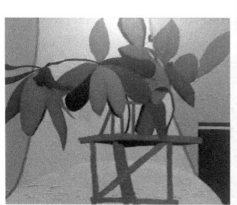
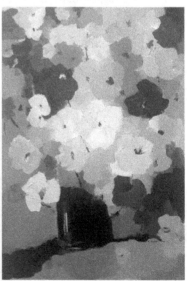

Paintings by my mother, Rosa Haber

My parents were the greatest people I have ever known, tenfold, but my life growing up was definitely not an episode of *Leave It to Beaver* or *Father Knows Best*. Granted, we had a big backyard to play in with apple, orange, and tangerine trees to climb, but if you look up the word "strict," you see my parents' pictures next to it. Today corporal punishment is grounds for a kind of punishment of its own, by the authorities; in those days it was not. At times a belt was used in our household. My mother used it very lightly but my father had other ideas, chasing me around our nineteen hundred square foot house on Fremont Street, in and out of its little warrens of rooms.

Physical punishment notwithstanding, I was not the most agreeable kid ever born. Brenda always did the right thing and got straight A's. Charlie played by the rules: he was a very cute kid and the proverbial "yes" man. I, on the other hand, was not all that adorable. I was obstinate, downright defiant, and even lazy, though strong lessons I'd come to learn about the repercussions of being lazy would lead me to where I am today, so I cannot fault the way I started out. If our lives indeed are scripted before we live them, and if this was my course, then quite simply this was my course. I was also addicted to baseball, watching incessantly on TV and playing, maybe since I was about four years old, and then at age seven in Little League. When I turned eight I was a starter—very young to be one but I was good at the game—and played first base. Our team was called the Navajos and believe it or not, I am still close friends with some of my teammates today: Bill Batey; Robert Batey; Ricky Guerra; and Robbie Freeman, who's an attorney here in Laredo. Let's face it, baseball is a universal language. We all spoke it and continue to. It'd be nothing for us to play from 6 a.m. to 6 p.m. during summer vacations. I just couldn't get enough. One day when I was about nine or ten I was running late for practice and, certain my mom was taking a nap, commandeered her car and drove myself to the ball park. A model kid I was not. Coach Chapman, who happened to be a Laredo-based FBI agent, was none too thrilled with me that day, I can assure you. Overall my obsession probably didn't thrill my family either, but little did I or anyone know that a dozen or so years down the road, baseball would turn out to be the key to a wholly unanticipated future. More on that later.

First, it's important to note that my father was a workaholic. I'm sure my work ethic comes from him, though it was no fun growing up essentially without him in the picture the way the other boys' fathers were. He typically put in sixteen- to eighteen-hour days, six days a week at the furniture store he owned, eventually opening more. I almost never saw him and he didn't attend any of my games which tended to hurt. On the other hand my mother, knowing nothing about the sport, always came.

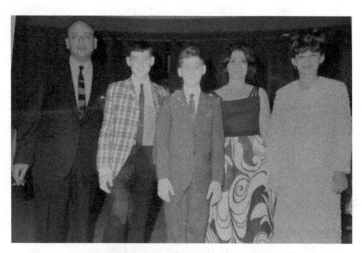

Left to right: My father, Maurice Haber, me, my brother
Charlie, my sister Brenda, and my mother

On a rare family getaway when I was eleven, the five of us flew to New York for my cousin Neil's bar mitzvah in Brooklyn, home of the legendary Brooklyn Dodgers. I clearly remember the details including that it was a Wednesday, the name of the airline was Braniff, and that there was sheeting rain all day. We flew from San Antonio to Dallas for the final connecting flight to JFK, sitting on the stormy tarmac for what seemed like a year. It was 2 a.m. when we finally landed, heading straight for the Concourse Plaza Hotel in Brooklyn which I found out was a block and a half from Dodger Stadium. *Dodger Stadium*? I thought I'd died and gone to heaven. Who needed sleep? Actually who needed air?

The next morning my father's sister Esther and her husband Morty greeted us in the lobby, with bar mitzvah boy cousin Neil and his brother Lyle. The adults were scrambling to do things in preparation for the service which was to occur the following evening. This was around the time I learned a number of Yankee teammates lived in the hotel—*the hotel where I was staying*! I recall being unable to see straight, parking myself squarely on a couch to lay in wait in case one of them passed through.

"Here's a pad for autographs, son," my mother said, lovingly handing me what I perceived as the equivalent of the velvet cloth that would receive the crown jewels. She always got me.

I didn't move from the lobby all day. My mother joked that even if a kidnapper came for me I'd find a way to evade him, unless I had at least one Yankee autograph, in which case I'd have achieved my greatest goal thus far in my young life and be happy to go.

Part of my adventure that day was seeing one of the most celebrated sports broadcasters in history climb out of a cab in front of the hotel just as my mother, Aunt Esther, and her family got into another. It was the famous Red Barber and I thought it was a sign: I was on my way to meeting some real Yankee gold if I could just sit there long enough. Who needed food or a bathroom break when the gates to nirvana were about to swing completely open?

After some time a tall, lanky, somewhat familiar face walked through the Concourse. I knew him as a ball player though couldn't immediately identify him. You would immediately recognize Mickey Mantle or Roger Maris, but I struggled with this one. I felt he was someone relatively new to the major leagues, and though I'd committed the rosters of multiple teams to memory thanks in part to my baseball card collection, I just couldn't put my finger on his name—except to recall him as a pitcher. Interestingly, I also recalled his stats: this pitcher had had a banner year, winning sixteen out of twenty games. *What was his name?* I strode up to him with my pad, respectfully asking for his autograph, which he readily accommodated. His signature would thaw my brain freeze. It turned out he was none other than Al Downing. Back on the couch, I must have stared at his name for two hours before the spell was broken by my family's return. But much to my disappointment, no one was all that impressed, except perhaps Uncle Morty who I'd always considered the reason I was so mesmerized by the sport. Whenever he came to visit us in Texas, he'd spend hours regaling me with stories and stats on what was clearly his passion too. I was never so happy to be a human sponge.

The next morning my dad took Brenda and Charlie on errands with Uncle Morty, telling me to stay behind with mom. I never minded spending time with her because I considered her totally cool. Growing up, she was both mother and father in the wake of an absentee spouse. Granted we always knew where dad was, toiling away at his furniture stores, but he wasn't with us. My cool mom let me run up and down the hallways while she took her time getting dressed for the important day ahead. Eventually we got into the elevator to go down, stopping to let someone in. My eyes bugged out of my head. Lightning had struck twice in one place. That someone was none other than Al Downing, and I introduced him my mother.

"Mom," I said, smiling so wide it hurt because I personally knew a sports celebrity, "this is Mr. Downing. He plays for the New York Yankees."

"Nice to meet you, Mr. Downing," my soon-to-be uncool mother replied in her distinct composite accent, "Exactly what position do you play?"

I was so embarrassed by her lack of knowledge of this Yankee Great's position and stature that I wanted to run away at ninety mph, but we were still descending. He was incredibly polite and unassuming, gently informing her he was a pitcher. When we got to the lobby he walked away, telling my mother how nice it was to meet her, that she had a very nice young boy, patting me on the head. As my mother smiled kindly in return for his compliment, in my usual way I kind of wanted to tell her where I thought she should go, and it was not to the first floor. I later realized what I perceived as my mother's imperfection was part of the beauty of who she was in regarding all people as equal, no one above anyone else.

"Mom!" I exclaimed a minute later when he was out of earshot, in eleven-year-old decibels I was fairly good at and possibly for all of Brooklyn to hear, "He's a *pitcher* for the *Yankees*!" She apologized profusely and again she was cool. She'd redeemed herself and I made sure to tell her it was okay. We loved each other more than life and sometimes the pain I feel when I think of her now is indescribable. I miss her every minute of every day.

If You Build It...

One summer I had a weekend paper route which required me to get up at 4 a.m. It required that my mother did as well, something she clearly didn't look forward to, but she'd do anything for me. She helped me fold all the papers and drove me around as I threw them at the wrong houses. That was the summer my friends and I also decided to take over an empty lot across from Ricky Guerra's house to build our own baseball field. My mom went to the owner of the Tumble In diner to see if they'd sponsor us with uniforms, or some semblance of them. They said yes and she ended up stapling the words "Tumble In" on the back of our shirts. The owner of the empty lot let us build a backstop and outfield fence. Summer temperatures are scorching in Texas and my mother used to wake me up very early to get out there before the sun bored a hole through my head. The mothers used to bring us lemonade as we wildly swung hammers and used all our strength and conviction to build our dream, painstakingly mowing the jagged, rock-strewn grass, until it was done. The thing is, we had our unofficial team, but we never played against anybody. We didn't care. All summer long we hit balls and had the time of our lives.

The whole time I was growing up my mother was with me, around me, supporting me. She came to all my games, bought milkshakes, took my brother and me swimming. The compassion she showed her children and I think especially me, more often than not the demon child, was limitless. She loved the living daylights out of us. There was a period of years when she took Brenda, Charlie, and me to Mexico for the summer to visit my grandparents. We'd ride horses and though her parents had strict rules about what we could and couldn't do in the house, I remember these times as something magical.

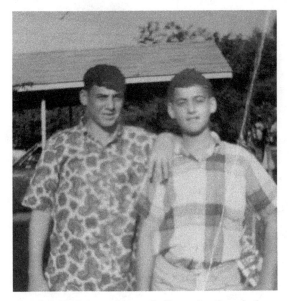

Charlie (right) with me (left) at the family house

When we didn't go to Mexico, and during the school year, with the exception of the occasional charred-beyond-recognition steak cookout on a Sunday, Saturdays were the only time I actually got to be around my father. My mother used to drop us off at the furniture store all day so she could have some quiet time, socialize with friends, and run her errands. I got to see this tall, formidable man in action and again I'm sure that's where my work ethic comes from as he never gave less than 150 percent. When I look back, though, as driven and successful as he was, I don't think he was ever truly happy. I'm sure he died a sad man, never getting to know who he was inside, and might have been, had he not been trying so hard not to be his father.

2

In the Clearing

"Sometimes the choice of professions picks us, not the other way around." – Anonymous

In the previous chapter, I mentioned my baseball obsession would lead to a completely unanticipated future. That future was medicine though the path was scarcely credible. The fact is the reason I didn't do very well in school was that I was a completely lazy kid. Consequently, the odds of my getting into and making it all the way through medical school, or even considering medical school in the first place were about a billion to one. But I did—on all counts.

First, I have a memory about my laziness. In fact I have many, but this one is worth sharing. One day I was riding in the car with my mother. I can't recall exactly where we were headed, but I happened to look down and see my fat stomach poking out of my light green shirt. I can see this as though it were yesterday. Granted, I did play baseball, so I moved my body at certain times of the year, but my mother also bought us a lot of milkshakes in those days as Laredo is hot as hell. What kid doesn't appreciate a sweet, cooling treat like that? Apparently, I appreciated them a little too much. I distinctly remember looking down, struck by what was sticking out of my obviously ill-fitting shirt. I probably just kept gaining weight and mom had to try and keep up with my ever-expanding girth. Even at age eight or nine, I considered my physical state a measure of the laziness of which I was becoming increasingly aware. While I didn't immediately act on my observation, the feeling was there and would rear its ugly head from time to time. But one day in a wholly unexpected way, and during March Madness—yes, I liked basketball too and had played a lot of pick-up games in school—the Fates took over and I finally did something about myself.

My path to medicine was through sports, but it wasn't a straight line. I've already established how much I love baseball, in fact fully participating in the sport until I was a freshman at the University of Houston. While there I dislocated my left knee sliding into home plate. My playing career was over, at least for a few years, and fortunately I was not there on a baseball scholarship. I could rely on my parents, and I also always had a job from the time I was in junior high school. In college I worked part time as an orderly in a very small, fifty-five bed hospital. Though I digress here for a minute, working in that environment was yet another example of my exposure to abject poverty. The patients were largely poor and marginalized. Most of the aides were tired, elderly Black women likely earning minimum wage, toiling away at these physically demanding, draining, unpleasant jobs for most of their lives. They didn't have a way out. I recall being asked by one of them to clean up a large pool of vomit in the hallway, realizing this is what she typically did day in and day out for decades.

In March of 1974, on spring break, I was in my Houston apartment watching a March Madness game on TV. The phone rang and I went to get it.

"Hey Milt!" The fiery Latin voice at the other end was vaguely familiar. "It's Roberto! Roberto Ramos! Remember?"

You could have knocked me over with anything. Here it was March Madness, and of all people, Roberto Ramos was calling. He was older, but he and I had been friends throughout school. He was maybe six foot two or a little taller and a star basketball player. We'd shot a lot of hoops together but I'd not heard from him in years.

"How are you doing? How's it all going? What's going on?" he asked, his earnest inquiry like that of a long lost brother. In fact he really was my Laredo brother.

I told him I was doing pretty well, vegging in front of a good game on TV. He told me he was in medical school in Monterrey, Mexico. One of seven children born to a struggling, exceedingly hard-working family, they barely got by the whole time we were growing up. I knew he was always trying to make something of himself, and this? Medical school? Wow, I thought. *Wow!*

"Let's get together," he said, to which I readily agreed. "I mean now," he added. "You can get a flight."

I don't know what possessed him to call me out of the blue like that, or even more unbelievably why I immediately booked a flight, but next thing I knew he was picking me up at the airport in Mexico—my mother's magnificent Mexico. We drove to his apartment, actually a miniscule rented room with a couple of fans, one of which was broken, and no air conditioning. It was 11 a.m. and he asked if I wanted to take a rest after my flight.

"Hell, no!" I said. I was truly impressed with the whole idea of his being in medical school and wanted to waste no time seeing the campus. We proceeded to the school, walking around as he pointed out various buildings, soon greeted by four or five guys he knew. They looked more American than anything else and I asked where they were from. I was right—all were from the US and all studying medicine there, including one from Houston where I was an undergrad or would be for two more months. The program was six years long and one of them commented that it was a fantastic school. To this day I'm not sure what happened but something turned over in me. The fact is I'd been applying to dental schools, and had been accepted, but the only reason I'd chosen that path was one of my many jobs in high school had been working for a dentist. He liked me, wrote a letter of recommendation, and pushed me in that direction. With nothing better to do that I could think of, I applied. But apparently something else was going on for me (the life script?) and I was going to pay attention.

Roberto suggested we do some bar hopping, perhaps meet some girls. It wasn't something I typically liked to do, preferring to be in bed early and saving my energy for daylight pursuits, but when in Rome, err, Monterrey. By 3 a.m. I'd had it, so we went back to his room. I'm an early riser and woke him four-and-a-half hours later, dragging him out for breakfast. It was a new day and as they say, time was a'wastin'. Over strong coffee and huevos rancheros, I told him I wanted to go back to the school.

"What? It's the weekend," he replied. "Let's have some fun."

"I'm serious," I told him. Mexico and everything in it was bursting with color, something my mother loved so much, including this bright little café. But in that moment it all disappeared—receded into the background. Except for the day in the Concourse Plaza Hotel lobby when Al Downing walked in, I was never so focused on anything in my life. Everything else kind of faded out. There was a clearing and I was standing in it. "I have to see your dean," I told Roberto, "the dean of the medical school."

It was Saturday but fortunately the dean was there. His office was two long blocks from the medical school and as always in Mexico it was hot, hot, hot, but I didn't feel it. The only things I saw—and felt deep inside of me—were the next steps for the path I was suddenly on. I practically ran the four flights up to his office. We knocked on the door and Roberto introduced me. I told him I was very impressed with my friend attending medical school, and impressed with the students I'd met the day before who'd told me how much they liked going to school there, and I wanted to matriculate. In impeccable English, the dean said he was very pleased to hear that.

"So what sport do you play?" he asked next, without hesitation. I looked at him, then at Roberto, then back at him.

"Ah, well, football of course," I lied. Clearly I was taken aback. Instead of inquiring about my grades, or interest in a specialty, or anything remotely related to grades or medicine, I was being asked about my athletic prowess. The reason I said football was because some of the Americans I'd met played for the school, or so Roberto had told me, and if the dean was asking I figured that would open the door.

He sent us off in the direction of Coach Cayetano. We climbed into Roberto's car, driving to the football field. An assistant coach told me to go inside the locker room, find a uniform, and change. Not being a player, Roberto was not allowed in, leaving me to struggle with the gear that was about to become more like an exit vehicle from my dream of medical school than a point of entry. I couldn't figure out how to wear it. Another team member named Robert "Beto" Villegas happened to walk in, asking me what position I played.

"Me? I'm a middle linebacker," I lied again. This time I don't know where that came from, but the next thing I knew he was walking me out onto the field to introduce me to the linebacker coach, though not before informing me I had the uniform on backwards. The helmet was also rocking all over the place. Most football players wear their gear like a second skin, which clearly I did not. I joined a bunch of linebackers, whereupon the coach instructed me to hit the practice dummy hard. Calling up everything I had I ran at full speed and hit it, nearly breaking my neck, landing backwards on the ground. The coach glared, standing over me, about to speak in perfect English. "You've never played an ounce of football in your life, have you, Haber." This time I could not tell a lie. "You're gonna' kill yourself out here," he continued. "I highly recommend you get off the field." The assistant coach came up and walked me over to Coach Cayetano, who'd been watching and had been informed about me.

"I hear you want to attend medical school," he said. I nodded sheepishly, wondering if my chances had just been obliterated. "I can do that for you, but it isn't going to be through football." I don't recall all the details but I must have done some talking that day, or perhaps my friend Roberto Ramos had said something directly to him, so Coach Cayetano knew about my baseball aptitude and long, proven history with the sport. "You can come here, but only if you play baseball for us," he said.

On Sunday morning I flew back to Houston. Spring break was over. I was so excited I hardly recall landing at Intercontinental Airport or the drive back to my apartment. Once inside, I grabbed the phone to call my mother, telling her dental school would never happen, but that I was going to medical school instead. Sorry if it sounds like a cliché, but it's the dream of Jewish mothers and fathers everywhere that their children become lawyers or doctors, and I was following suit—not so much for them, but for me. I figured they'd be proud.

The interesting thing about my parents, and though my mother was always demonstrably affectionate, is that they never gave the three of us much in the way of direction. A form of tough love? Perhaps. I'm not sure, but I do have some thoughts here on the matter.

Throughout my upbringing I was always searching for myself... trying to find out who I was. I'm sure a lot of people do that, but I can recall my quest starting at a very, very young age. Even today, with all I've accomplished and with the path I'm on in medical research, I'm still searching. How can I do more? How can I expand the research I've undertaken? This is something I ask myself all the time, and then again and again and yet again, much to the frustration of those closest to me professionally! I tend to be relentless, the button that gets stuck in the on position.

As a child, my father wouldn't help me in my search. My mother wouldn't help me either. She nurtured me, and of course they fed me, but the message I always got was you have to find yourself in your own way. They relied on my sister, brother, and me to make our own decisions, forge our own paths, dig ourselves out of any holes in which we'd find ourselves as a result, and make a course correction. We had to learn to choose what was right and wrong for ourselves; they were never going to do that for us. I think it was tough on me at times, but as I grew I understood they wanted us to become the individuals we had it within ourselves to become, not overly influenced by who they were as a result of their life experiences and what they wanted for us. When you really think about it, they didn't choose the easy way when raising us. Sure, there was discipline, but I'm sure there were many other instances when they had to restrain themselves, such as when we were making mistakes or being unreasonable and when what they really wanted to do was pick us up by the ears and drop us squarely in the middle of the right course. But they didn't. They left that up to us.

My mother, having fled Eastern Europe, was fiercely Jewish. She reveled in her heritage. She wasn't orthodox but a willing adherent to her faith. Yet she never imposed it on me, instead deciding that while she wanted me to have a sense of our family's heritage, it wasn't imperative for me to embrace it wholeheartedly as she did. That was a good thing for me as frankly I felt disconnected from it. My friends were Black, white, Latino, and all different faiths with only some being Jewish. Also Laredo is 90 percent Hispanic so clearly my family was in the minority. That's how I grew up and all I knew, and I was fine with it.

Medical school in Monterrey was my choice, and—yes—of all things baseball had gotten me in. It's true my parents were proud but possibly not in the way other Jewish parents would have been, like it was the only option for a life well lived. This is no offense to those who still subscribe to that way of thinking. I knew they wanted the best for me no matter what life choices I was going to make. I guess it didn't hurt, though, that this was the road I was choosing. I could do a lot worse.

My big sister Brenda was always an overachiever. She eventually obtained her Ph.D. in psychology and has a thriving clinical practice in

Seattle. Back in high school, she decided, with my parents' endorsement, to leave Laredo for a better education at St. Mary's Hall, a private boarding school in San Antonio. She was always the family scholar and in that respect I always had some pretty big shoes to fill along the way, but my decision to go to medical school wasn't made in the realm of competition or shoe-filling. The only thing I can surmise is that it was a calling much in the way years later my transitioning into research and clinical trials, while maintaining my private practice, was an extension of that calling. Or, in further dissecting things, perhaps research is where I was always meant to be, in order to help more people than I could in private practice, but could never do it without first becoming a doctor. I cannot emphasize enough what my having the privilege to be in medical research, executing clinical trials, means to me at this time in the course of world events—what it *feels* like—except maybe to equate it with the following experience.

In 1962, my family was driving back from California on one of the few family vacations we ever took. I recall the year vividly because we were listening to the car radio, hearing that Marilyn Monroe had just died. Reentering Texas, we came upon Big Bend National Park—which to a kid looks like billions of acres, though technically it is 801,163 acres. To a ten-year-old boy this was a giant outdoor canvas to paint. Suddenly my dad announced we were getting out and going horseback riding. I thought my heart would rocket straight out through my chest—it was a real high. I'd ridden a few times when visiting my maternal grandparents in Mexico; I loved it beyond anything and never wanted to get off.

My mother had never been on a horse in her life. That day she had on a dress—the fluffy, billowing kind women wore in the era. I always thought she looked beautiful but she was clearly concerned, saying she was not getting on a horse. My dad insisted, and if I've not said it before, or enough, she was wholly devoted to him. He was not an easy man yet throughout their marriage she supported and catered to his every wish and whim. He went to the trunk, opened a suitcase, and pulled out a pair of his giant brown pants. Dad was six feet tall. Mom was not, and they were probably five times her size, but she put them on and off we went. I remember my mother kind of choking and gagging in the wind, her hair twisting and turning like a tornado around her face as we galloped along rugged terrain that, at least to me, was the stuff of paradise. Those four or five hours together passed in a heartbeat. That was the closest I'd ever felt as a family. It was our best life possible. Unfortunately, it was an experience that, because of my father's work life, would never be repeated. But now, in a sense, I feel the same kind of joy—almost a high, if you will, in regard to my role in medical research, helping ensure other families get to live their best lives possible too.

3

In the Thick of It

"There are no shortcuts to anyplace worth going." -Hellen Keller

A 1973 movie based on the John Jay Osborn novel, *The Paper Chase,* followed a student's arduous journey through the first year of law school. There's a scene that involves throwing up after class in the bathroom, something I wanted to do many times in my first, second, third, fourth, fifth, and sixth years of medical school, and particularly when it was all over. Let me explain.

In 1980, following graduation, I drove home to Laredo to await the results of my Educational Commission for Foreign Medical Graduates, or ECFMG. These boards would determine if I got an internship and residency in the United States, in short, if I ever got to practice medicine in my native country. In addition to all my classes and rotations, I literally studied for it day and night for an entire year. The possibility that I'd fail plagued me in the weeks that followed, so much so that I literally lay in the middle of my parents' living room carpet, paralyzed by levels of fear and anxiety I'd never known before. I call them "buzz brain" anxiety attacks. It wasn't so much that I needed not to fail for my parents' sake, though that was certainly part of it. Paramount to that was the pivotal moment in a Mexican café where I'd set my sights on a different life, a life I wanted to see through. I *had* to see it through without failure. Medical school required a level of discipline I wasn't sure I had, though I'd certainly found it and for that reason also I had to succeed. Though crashing and burning was a looming possibility, I had too much invested for that kind of outcome. To quote a line from another popular movie, 'failure was not an option'. After more than twenty years of lazing, loafing, and coasting, and even to a large extent squandering away my college years in Houston dating and goofing off because studying was like leprosy to me, the moment of truth had occurred over a plate of eggs in Mexico. I couldn't imagine throwing away six grueling years of my life. But had I passed or failed?

The fact is I'd joined Roberto on that fateful weekend in 1974 on a whim. I thought we were going to goof around, meet girls, and have a blast. But there it was: my future put in motion by a call from an old friend. Accepted to medical school, I drove down in late June or early July of that year. I didn't want to live with Roberto because he had a reputation as a playboy and I was about to become the most serious, studious, do or die person I'd ever known. I moved into a large apartment with four Americans, all from New York, who went to Universidad de Monterrey medical school, a private university Roberto attended. I would be attending Universidad Autónoma de Nuevo Leon—a state school, however—but the whole sports thing connected the schools and Nuevo Leon was the school that issued my baseball scholarship. One of my roommates, Carlos, was a New York engineer of Cuban nationality who'd decided to change careers at age forty-eight. I was a bit jealous of him because somehow he'd gotten the biggest room, but boy did I learn a lot from him about work ethic. My room was like a closet, once the maid's room. It was away from everybody which really allowed me to study my ass off once I closed the door. During winter months the room was so cold and damp I got a hold of some carpeting from my father's furniture store and covered the whole floor, which helped a little. I also got an air conditioner for the heat, which was most of the time. This was no Taj Mahal but I was comfortable enough.

I went to my classes and buried myself in the books fifteen or more hours a day. This was broken down into alone hours plus my study group at night, comprised of my apartment mates. Classes were in Spanish but I got the books in English. Fortunately I'd been raised by a Spanish-speaking mother so I had a slight advantage over many other foreign students, but nothing was easy. By the same token I was so focused not even a natural disaster could have pried me away from my goal of making it all the way to graduation. I feared failure, deciding if I couldn't make it in medical school I just wouldn't make it anywhere. It was the ultimate test. I studied and prayed—prayed that I'd pass pathology, anatomy, physiology, pharmacology. The challenges didn't end, the pressure never letting up day in and day out for six years, including a year of nationally mandated primary care social service, or *pasantia*, for the country's underserved communities. Overall I think it was the most focused I've ever been in my life.

Though I was clearly in a vise for six straight years, I must say the *pasantia* year was an experience I will never forget and sometimes long for again in my dreams. I could have avoided it altogether by taking something called the Fifth Pathway, which many Americans elect to do in order to get back into the US and practice medicine at that point, but I didn't feel I was equipped to take that exam. I had signed up for the whole Mexican medical school experience and the *pasantia* was part of it, in fact something similar, I would think, to the mandatory year of military service for Israeli students. My study group as a whole concurred about taking on this kind of field work and each of us geared up to do our part.

There are choices for the *pasantia*, such as working as a doctor on a large ranch or in a small town, even in the poorest parts of a big city, etc. I chose a small town of eleven hundred people about thirty miles north of Monterrey called General Escobedo—now actually incorporated into the city itself as Monterrey has grown. For every moment of challenge in this town there was a moment of magic—maybe more magic than challenge. It would never have happened had I attended medical school in the US, and when I think about the things to be most grateful for in my life, this always rises to the top.

My office was in a clinic attached to the local elementary school. Office hours were from 9 to 11 a.m., and 1 to 3 p.m., Monday through Friday. A block away was a convenience store owned by a family to whom I became quite attached. I'm not sure if they felt sorry for this earnest Young Turk or possibly some respect for the way I was able to care for members of their community, but they fed me well and always welcomed me with open arms like one of their own.

There were neither phones nor TVs in General Escobedo. Around the corner from the convenience store was a telegraph office, and I also became friendly with the young man who operated it. In slow times for me or when the clinic was closed midday, we'd sit in tall chairs outside, shooting the bull, just like a lazy afternoon scene out of *Andy of Mayberry*. I became friendly with the mayor, city leaders, and others of that ilk. Seems as though wherever I went, there was a pervading warmth and great lack of pretense in General Escobedo, something one might be hard pressed to find in the US.

At times during this externship things were quite exciting and at others a little boring. If no one came to see me during office hours, I was all alone. I had a supervisor that I never saw, and frankly, though the *pasantia* is designed to fulfill a vital service, there are reports that cite social service physicians are typically unpracticed, unsupervised, and unsupported. Significant demotivation, absenteeism, and underperformance typically plague the social service year.[1] Given my own circumstances, I could absolutely see how this was true, but I wasn't about to perform inadequately despite the absence of any leadership. My patients, albeit crushingly poor, deserved the same consideration and opportunity for good health as their wealthy and middleclass counterparts in other areas of the country. I learned before I got there that an average of three or four patients a day were seen by doctors who passed through. I was able to see fifteen a day. I treated everything from acute asthma to bronchitis. I started intravenous and Theophylline drips. I delivered babies in homes with dirt floors. It was interesting for me to see how quickly some of them came out, almost no labor involved, born to mothers who had delivered ten, fifteen, even twenty children ahead of them.

With all of its obvious challenges and limitations, that year in General Escobedo was one of the best years of my life, so much so that I considered extending my stay. I earned a paltry thousand pesos a month, the equivalent of a few US dollars, but I never felt richer.

As my *pasantia* came to an end, members of the town came by to thank me and see me off, gifting me with a horse, a cow, and pigs. You can't refuse or it is considered an insult, and even more than that this was the ultimate expression of their gratitude—something I did not take lightly. I was moved beyond anything, especially when they

---

[1] Andrew Van Wieren, et al. Service, training, mentorship: first report of an innovative education-support program to revitalize primary care social services in Chiapas, Mexico. Nov. 3, 2014. Extracted April 30, 2021. NCBI Resources. https://www.ncbi.nlm.nih.gov/pmc/articles/PMC4220002/

brought out the cake! Fortunately I was able to give the animals to a fellow medical school student whose parents had a farm on the outskirts of Monterrey.

Looking back, I can honestly say this was the year in my life when I really, truly felt as though I belonged somewhere. The people of Mexico are beautiful people. They are warm-hearted and hard working. They are big believers in God. They carry their lives through faith, and you feel it every day as they tell you *vaya con Dios*, or go with God. I sometimes thought about what my mother experienced coming in from a bleak and somber Poland, and I knew it was absolutely true what she felt about this place and these people. I've traveled to many places but Mexico is unlike any other in the world. Inherent in Mexican culture is a profound grace, acceptance, generosity, and a genuine joy of community—increasingly rare qualities I've yet to find in other societies.

Artificial Means

In terms of my coursework, anatomy was probably the hardest. We had to learn everything in Spanish which I translated to English. But there was also Latin terminology which tripped me up, navigating from one language to another and to another.

The night before a pharmacology exam I was struggling to understand and then memorize everything I needed to. For some reason I found it hard to focus, likely nerves and exhaustion, feeling as though I was all over the place like a leaky bottle of syrup. I couldn't get it together. A member of my study group took me aside.

"I want you to take this," he said. I recall his hand opening to reveal something shiny. Amphetamines. "It'll wake you up," he continued. "You can focus."

I stared momentarily at the panacea in his palm, telling him I didn't want to take anything like that. "Just take it," he said. "Do you want to pass or fail? It will make a difference."

At that point I weakened. It was hard to argue the point. I was not feeling like myself and terrified of failing. Reluctantly I took it, returning to my tiny room to study some more. Within ten minutes the words on the page lifted up, heading straight into my eyes. I totally freaked out, running to find the "perpetrator" who chuckled, reassuring me I was going to be all right. "Uh-huh. This means you are focused," was all he said.

The next morning at 8 a.m., I sat down to take the exam and aced it. The irony was not lost on me that pharmaceuticals helped me pass a pharmacology exam. Though the pressures of surviving medical school more commonly than not lead students to artificial means, I never took a pill like that again. In fact I've never smoked and don't even drink. I don't apologize for my actions that day because I need to take full responsibility for making the kind of decision I did, but as a rule I just don't believe in it for myself. At one point I considered going into psychiatry, a specialty where medication is warranted, liberally prescribed, and in some cases life-changing for patients who cannot function normally without it. But I could not see spending my entire medical career prescribing and adjusting diets of narcotics and antidepressants at fifteen-minute intervals, the length of time many psychiatry appointments last today. And psychiatry is a never ending, revolving door of unfortunate bipolar issues and depression. I had my psychiatry rotation and many of the patients were suffering from psychosis—just couldn't comprehend what was going on around them or what I was saying. I felt unable to connect. No offense to the field, but through trial and error I've found I am much more hands on, needing more immersion in my patient's lives, and more give and take to help them achieve the best outcomes.

Of Baselines and Bovines

I'd been accepted to Universidad Autónoma de Nuevo Leon on a baseball scholarship. As much as I needed to study, in baseball season the effort I put into sports was equally matched in terms of discipline. At the same time, I didn't want to sacrifice a moment more away from my studies than I had to. When the team took a bus for away games, a round trip that could result in as many as sixteen hours on the road, I elected to fly. But on shorter trips I took the team bus, winding through boisterous cities or serene countryside. I'd seen some of Mexico when my mother took us to the grandparents' house in summer, but now I got to see a whole lot more of what had given her absolute joy from the moment her ship docked in Veracruz forty years earlier.

I recall one away game in particular about twenty miles outside of Monterrey. When we got to the playing field, we were greeted by cows and dirt. Lots of dirt, in fact, and no grass. Not much in the way of baseball accoutrements, just cow patties. When the game started, they simply moved the cows off to the side so we could play. Putting this into perspective, I'd never have had this kind of experience playing ball in the US. The opposing pitcher was no more than fourteen, maybe even younger. In Central America and Mexico, the *prepatoria*, something like our high school, starts at about that age and then at sixteen they go to college, or directly to medical school without college. It wasn't uncommon for the teams we played against to have younger team members, and let me tell you, this kid had a left-handed fast ball like I've never seen and may not see again in my lifetime. I told him to save his arm. I wasn't sure how he'd come to the attention of a baseball scout but over the years others had, including Fernando Valenzuela, Beto Avila, Aurelio Rodriguez, Jorge Orta, and more. I knew if he could do it, he'd have a serious future. I never forgot that arm!

Home Again

Hitting the books 24/7, and throughout my requisite rotations and the internships and residency that would follow (please see chapter 4), I would get closer and closer to choosing internal medicine for myself. Internal medicine is something like being a private investigator, getting a patient history but then trying to piece together what's going on which isn't always obvious. It's what I call an investigative science. Every day is beset by new challenges where years of experience increasingly pay off. You try to analyze the symptoms, and sometimes what the patient is not aware of or even not telling you for one reason or another, to get to the root of the problem. I can't see practicing any other kind of medicine.

As I started to recount at the beginning of the chapter, after six long years of medical school, graduation finally came. When I took the ECFMG, I was the last one to leave the room. My buddies from our study group were waiting for me outside, and I told them I flunked the s**t out of it. *I was that sure.*

My parents had moved from Fremont Street where we grew up to Belmont Street into a really nice home. But it could have been a cell for all I knew. I hardly noticed. The walls were closing in on me. In the weeks I waited for news of a pass or fail, I honestly thought I was going crazy. I remember lying down in the living room where my parents and I were watching television and though I didn't confide anything to them, my entire life collapsed into a little ball. That's the best way for me to describe the terror that gripped me every waking hour and even in my sleep. A residency had to come next, but if I couldn't work in the US, what then?

When the results finally came by mail you could have heard me shout all the way back to Monterrey—and General Escobedo. In time I would learn only six or seven out of three hundred fifty who took the boards passed; my entire study group among them.

4

In the Process

"Two roads diverged in a wood and I—I took the one less travelled by, and that has made all the difference." -Robert Frost

We have a close-knit family, and the opportunity to stay with my cousins Michael and Jake Kukoff in New York City was a big help while I looked for a residency. Ahead of that, a med school friend named Serapio Vela and his girlfriend lived a couple of blocks from LaGuardia Airport, so when I first flew to New York, I bunked with them for a few days while I got my bearings. I was fortunate to be able to rely on people who cared about me in my life.

I didn't do the match, a more traditional approach where you apply to different residencies around the country, identifying your first, second, and third choices. A lot of people from my medical school in Mexico didn't do it either. I preferred instead to pound the pavement and get a firsthand look at the facilities where I might be working before committing to anything.

I applied the same diligence to this task that I'd called up in school, making this time really count, going everywhere. I visited hospitals in Syracuse, Rochester, Queens, and New Jersey. I was accepted to many but was glad I'd taken the time to explore them as some were in such shocking condition I'd have been in shock myself from my first day of work forward. The last thing I needed was more anxiety. I had my eye on Cabrini Medical Center, now defunct but founded in 1973: a merger of two Manhattan hospitals. Named for a revered Catholic nun, Mother Frances Xavier Cabrini (now canonized), I figured it couldn't hurt. But I was not accepted there. I was, however, accepted to Beekman Downtown Hospital where I first did a term of volunteering—a pre-internship opportunity. The first year of the three-year residency that follows is typically considered the internship.

At Beekman Downtown, the majority of patients were Asian, routinely utilizing our staff interpreters. The staff had a global diversity of its own, ranging from Chinese to Russian to German to Czechoslovakian, with my chief resident an aggressive, imposing, often intimidating six-foot tall Russian female. Had it been another era, she'd probably have succeeded as a spy or in law enforcement, as tangling with her was not a good idea.

Beekman Downtown was an extremely busy place. As an intern I put in Foley catheters, started IVs, took patients downstairs for radiology, and so much more. I was required to do a lot of hands-on work and though at first it was daunting, I got my feet wet very quickly or to use another cliché, it was clearly a baptism by fire. I used to observe nurses doing a lot of charting but not much more. The emergency room was total chaos. You would try to get a history on a patient who didn't speak English, flagging down an interpreter, all while being repeatedly poked in the shoulder by colleagues who needed your help—stat. It was sheer madness.

Criticism was hurled at us freely; sometimes I wished I were invisible or could find a corner in which to hide to avoid it, because it could be utterly humiliating. I recall one patient brought in for pneumonia. I was standing there to give my superiors the morning report. They were demanding urinalysis numbers first, and besides being incredulous at this, I was a smartass.

"The patient has *pneu-mo-nia*," I said, the emphasis not missed in my protracted pronunciation of the word.

"I don't care what he has," was the stern retort. "We want the urinalysis."

If you read the *New England Journal of Medicine*, no matter what the disease, urinalysis is presented first. The hospital was following protocol, and I was expected to know the lab work essentially by memory before presenting it. This was quite a humbling experience, to say the least. I felt like a tiny insignificant bug that day but never repeated my mistake. I had superiors covering me, but they weren't really covering my back. Bottom line is it was I who needed to have the back of the patients in my care. I learned it was not acceptable to punt or bullshit your way around Beekman, something that has continued to serve me every day of my life, professional or otherwise. If you're not all in, you'd better get out.

Toward the end of my internship I got a call from my sister Brenda, who lived in Dallas with her husband and two little boys. Brenda and I got busy with our own lives over the years but managed to maintain a nice relationship. She was in a pinch, her husband interviewing for an IT job in Miami, and she needed me to fly down and babysit. As I've said a dozen times, I think there's a life script out there because had she not called and had I not been sitting in an airport waiting for a flight to Dallas, I'd probably not have been reading a particular issue of the *New England Journal of Medicine*. I happened to flip to the back of the issue to check out open residencies. With hot weather in my blood, I wasn't thrilled to be in New York with its bone chilling winters of which I'd already suffered through two. One time I'd gone to a Dunkin' Donuts a block away from my cousins Michael and Jake's apartment, where I was staying. I was headed downtown and Jake uptown, and we often did this together to grab something on our way. I bought a lemon-filled donut and by the time I'd walked a few blocks it was all but frozen. I chucked it in a trash can, shivering the rest of the way to work as usual.

In the Dallas airport, I scanned the back of *NEJM*. A one-year opportunity at the Veterans Affairs Medical Center at Marshall University jumped out at me. Located in Huntington, West Virginia, at least it would be somewhat warmer. I ran to a payphone and by the end of the conversation, they'd asked to interview me the following Monday—three days hence. Instead of reporting for work at Beekman, I made some excuse about being stuck in Dallas and flew into a small airport on the Kentucky/West Virginia border, appearing front and center for my interview at the appointed time. I met the head of the department who must have liked me; I was offered the job the same day. I couldn't have been more relieved to be leaving NYC, though the universe was about to shake it up for me one more time as I've learned it often does when people are on the brink of a huge transition.

A week or so before I left, I bought a Nissan 240z for the drive to West Virginia. A new job and a new life warranted new wheels (why not!), and though I didn't have a lot of money, I wanted to do this for myself. I went out the morning I was to leave and it was gone—just like that. New York hospitality. Thankfully I'd sold my old Mustang to someone I knew, for a thousand dollars, and when I called him about the situation he was only too pleased to sell it back to me though for a two hundred dollar profit—lest I forget I was in New York. Had cousin Michael not fronted me the twelve hundred dollars, I have no idea how I'd have made it to Huntington. In reality I did have mixed feelings about leaving New York because my cousins were very, very good to me. In fact they were nothing short of great the whole time I was there, but somewhere in my bones I felt it was time to move on.

Marshall Law

Despite being ready for a change, I wasn't sure what to expect at Marshall University or in West Virginia for that matter. An apartment complex about twenty miles away from the hospital appealed to me, a little far out from where I'd like to have been, but it was brand new and I liked the look of it. It was a nice place to come home to, especially because it was about to turn into a very, very tough year. It wasn't so much about medicine, but the personalities with whom I worked were different than my colleagues and even my supervisors in New York. Given New York's reputation, you'd think it'd be the opposite but it surely wasn't. Residents at Marshall were tougher and more distant, but I kept in mind the university had one of the most celebrated infectious disease departments and a very fine cardiology department. I was trying to absorb as much as I could. The residency program was small which has advantages because you don't get swallowed up, yet you don't necessarily get the exposure and opportunities you might in a larger program.

My first night on call I was assigned to the ICU. Soon I was told to take a patient from the emergency room upstairs to the unit, however the ER doctor threw a thousand directions at me, none of which I understood. He alternately rambled and spoke a million miles a minute and I got possibly one out of every five words. I was completely lost, and here's my patient, only a forty-five year old intubated male with a myocardial infarction in cardiogenic shock. I was in shock myself, frantically searching for my chief resident who was nowhere to be found. This man could die on my watch, and I didn't know what to do. An ICU nurse caught a glimpse of the sorry sight I apparently was and offered to step in. She knew I was incredibly frightened.

"We're going to have to put a Swan Ganz in the patient," she said quietly. Though she couldn't have been kinder to me, as with the ER doctor, I had no idea what she was saying.

"A catheter to measure pressure in the heart," she explained.

"Who puts it in?" I asked.

"That would be you," she replied.

I told her I'd never before done this and she assured me she'd guide me. It was about 9 p.m. and it took my shaky hands and even shakier brain an hour to complete the procedure. In time I'd be able to do it in ten minutes, but not on that formidable night when I lost my Swan Ganz catheter virginity. Around 3 or 4 a.m. my chief resident happened to run into me, asking for an update on all my admitted patients. He spied the Swan Ganz monitor and asked who put in the device. I told him I'd done it, and he proceeded to ask me what the PA pressure was. Well, there it was again. I had no idea how to gauge PA—or pulmonary artery—pressure. I'd read something about it but that had been the extent of things. Anyway he was fairly impressed, and I never forgot the woman who saved my proverbial ass that night, in fact keeping in touch with her for years as she became a travelling nurse and took a well-deserved retirement in Miami.

The Resident Also Rises

In March of 1984, just before the end of my year-long internship, my chief of service said he wanted me to call a certain doctor at Ohio Valley Medical Center in Wheeling. OVMC was about three and a half hours northeast of Huntington, forty miles from Pittsburgh. He supplied me with letters of recommendation and I was able to finish out the remaining two years of a requisite three-year medical residency in Wheeling. I was really glad I could. This was more of a community hospital, but the residency program was actually larger than the one from which I'd come and for its size a lot more collegial in attitude. I was far more comfortable. In my first year of the two I was interested in cardiology, the OVMC department being very strong. There were many professors I got to know well, some of whom would later attend my wedding, but first things first.

The first thing I noticed was their genuine investment in helping me develop as a good physician. The other residents—some in their forties and fifties—came from all over: South Carolina; Texas; Argentina; Cuba. The multicultural aspect was interesting and the underlining objective was for everyone to succeed and not compete against one another. We all jumped on the same bandwagon.

Socially, things were even more interesting as you'd be invited over to someone's apartment for Argentinian food one night and someone else's for Cuban on the next, and maybe out for burgers the next. There was interaction on all fronts; we were a close group. In New York, you'd leave the hospital for the night and that was it. I found most people cold—just like the winters. And while things weren't always easy in West Virginia, certainly not at my first hospital experience, nevertheless I just felt better once I got to Wheeling.

With that there were always challenges, only the further along I went in my residency, I noticed they were happening more to the younger ones coming up behind me. Whew! One day a second-year resident was learning how to put in central lines. As a senior resident, I explained that you put the line in an internal jugular in a specific hole at the side of the neck. Instead of going into the vein, he went into the artery, opening the syringe. Blood shot up to the ceiling. I'd turned around momentarily to get something for him to pass the catheter into the internal jugular, suddenly hearing a thud. He'd fainted. As I put some pressure on the artery, the more composed patient turned and asked me if the doctor was all right.

I'd thought about remaining in Wheeling after my residency was over and was offered a couple of positions, but in actuality salaries were tragically low. I figured I'd make more waiting tables in a nice restaurant than I would as a practicing physician, and I wasn't too far off. Cardiology required a fellowship anyway, and I never got around to doing it, but it bears mentioning that something like a month or two into my time at OVMC I had a patient code. Flatline. Asystole: no electrical activity in the heart. There are a group of people who immediately assemble around a code: nurses; charge nurse; phlebotomist—all have their duties in light of what's happening. I told one nurse to zap the patient, in other words give him an electroshock conversion—use the paddles—and she looked at me somewhat perplexed. I should have known this was a term used back in New York, or at least at Beekman, and used proper medical terminology as time was running out for the patient. It turned out he was fine as not more than a few seconds passed after the miscommunication where we took appropriate action. It could have been funny under different circumstances. A year later, I'd marry the nurse.

When Milton Met Rita

While our meeting was less than auspicious, it was something else I chalk up to meant to be. But first, we had some obstacles to overcome, such as finding a rabbi and a priest to perform a mixed marriage ceremony which forty years ago was even more of a challenge than it might be today. The first priest we approached told Rita not to marry me. We proceeded to visit the rabbi in Wheeling who I knew from my time there, but he also admonished us about intermarrying. Daunted and wondering what to do, I happened to mention it to a friend at the gym who told me about a Pennsylvania rabbi he thought might consider it. Uniontown was thirty minutes away, just over the border, so I called and he invited us to meet with him. In fact his response was so positive, so fast, it left me wondering what was wrong here. It wasn't long before I found out.

We got to the synagogue and the rabbi took us on a tour. We thanked him but said we didn't want to get married in Uniontown. As we were leaving, he said location wasn't an issue and he'd be pleased to perform the ceremony anywhere, quoting us the exorbitant sum of fifteen hundred dollars. Today, the average cost of a wedding officiant is around three hundred dollars, give or take. This was 1986, so it would have been a portion of that. I'd call him nothing short of mercenary, but our only option if we wanted a religious ceremony. Rita's mother had a connection in the Catholic Church and secured a priest that way. We set the date: August 16th. One hundred fifty people attended coming from points North, South, East, and West: Rita's and my families; friends; fellow medical students; doctors who'd guided me through my residency. Later someone asked if I was going to invite Al Downing. I probably would have if I'd had his telephone number, but frankly I was more focused on how I was going to earn a living at that point. The reception was held at a beautiful venue at Wheeling's historic 1,650-acre Oglebay Park, and Rita and I started our life together.

I spent eight or nine months working at various hospitals, focusing to some extent on emergency rooms to get trauma center experience. I knew at that point I wanted to specialize in internal medicine, but soaking up all that was available was only going to serve me in the long run. One day I got a call from my old friend Serapio Vela, in whose La Guardia Airport-adjacent apartment I'd spent a few days when I first landed in New York. He was finishing his surgical residency in Chicago. We'd more or less kept in touch and he asked if I'd consider joining him in a practice we'd form together in Corpus Christi. Go home to Texas? Sounded good to me! My parents had their home in Laredo, but also one as it turned out in Corpus Christi where my dad had opened one of his furniture stores. I called mom and said Rita and I were going to fly down to Corpus next weekend. Time has a way of erasing some of the fine details, but somehow when I was there Serapio and I got into a squabble about something. We had differences in the way we approached and structured things. I'd had hopes this would be a very good opportunity and felt deflated for a couple of days. Sitting around the dinner table with my parents and Rita, I came to the decision I was going to bail before I got deeper in with Serapio and it became harder to extricate myself from a partnership. I said I'd return to Wheeling where I'd had a few job offers.

"Milton," my mom said in a moment of motherly reckoning. "You're here in Texas. Why not go back home to Laredo for a few days and see how it feels? I'll bet the medical community would be interested in you, being a native son and all."

Her logical thinking stopped me in my tracks. Once again she had my back. The next day, Rita and I set off for Laredo, a city that impressed her with its rich cultural heritage and proximity to Mexico. First stop was Doctor's Hospital, a venue I'd helped build with my own hands the summer I worked construction. Seems growing up I was always working one job or another, and now I wondered if there might be a possibility I'd get to walk the corridors of this building as a physician. In a million years, who'd have ever thought it?

I met with the CEO, a Cuban gentleman named Dominiche. It didn't take long and he put a contract in front of me. He wrote down one hundred seventy-five thousand dollars, saying it wasn't official but that was the number he was thinking, plus living expenses. Dominiche also told me they'd cover my office rent for a year. In Virginia, one of my offers was for thirty thousand dollars, all in, and all I could think was holey moly (I'm tempering my usual vernacular here). The adjacent building where I'd have my practice was still in the construction stages, but it wouldn't be more than a few months before I could move in.

The thing is, high as I was (who needed amphetamines!), all of it sounded too good to be true. I didn't waste a minute contacting an attorney, Robert McCarthy, I knew back in Wheeling—someone who'd represented me in a lawsuit when I'd ruptured my Achilles tendon requiring surgery. I ended up dropping the suit, but we became friends. In this life, you just never know what's really intended when you first meet someone. Often it's not what it seems in the beginning. I was fortunate to have him in my circle. He reviewed the contract immediately, saying it looked legitimate. Everything was in order and he advised me to take it. Rita and I returned to Wheeling to pack up. She was pregnant with our son Paul at that point, and we were excited about starting our family in the environment where I'd grown up. I was understandably nervous about opening a practice, wanting all my ducks in a row. As the saying goes, I didn't know what I didn't know and didn't want to make mistakes. Through some networking, I found a consultant in Chicago—an expert on starting a medical practice. I drove from Wheeling to the Windy City where he and I convened for four days, hammering out all the details. I was confident it was going to be done right. He would join me in Laredo in a month when my doors were closer to opening.

I couldn't wait to get home to Laredo after that where Rita and her sister were already in a hotel waiting for me. It was July and I recall the temperature being something in the vicinity of one hundred fourteen degrees. Though Rita liked the area, she was not prepared for heat like that and being in an expectant state didn't help. Still, in view of the kind of life that lay ahead for us, she made a concerted effort.

So much of our journey is about the choices we make. I call this "brain making": part upbringing; part education; part socializing; etc. Not necessarily in that order, but the brain takes a bit out of each component and puts it all together in a perfect dish. Okay, not always perfect and certainly not always appealing, but it's all together. And it's all essential. It's also just part of a larger thing, as I believe there's a greater being that helps set the direction of our lives and gets us where we want to go. When I was young, I was anything but spiritual. Perhaps it's age or life experience, fortune or misfortune, health or illness such as my bout with COVID that determine one's growth and development in this realm. I've been told science—the basis of medicine—and spirituality don't mix, that they are strange bedfellows. But I have a king-sized bed with plenty of room for both.

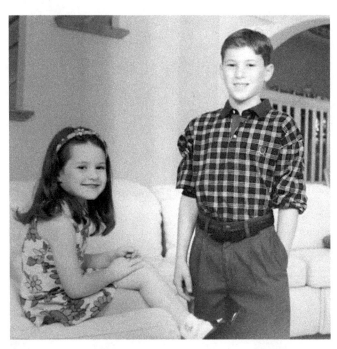

My children, Mariellen and Paul Haber, when they were little, both of them born and raised in Laredo.

5

In the ACTS

"Going on a retreat made me understand that I am on a journey with God, no different from anyone else."

- Milton Haber, M.D.

In addition to my mother who steered me back to Laredo, there are a few people in this world who've had my back for as many years as I can remember—even longer than I think I've had theirs. For Stella Alvarez, my medical receptionist, our decades-long relationship is as close as it gets to heavenly, or an other-worldly office experience. Her memory after all these years for specific people and events is remarkable, and for that reason she has helped me write this chapter. There are also things she wanted to include which I'd have chosen to leave out because in a way they embarrass me, but they are here anyway. I know I am a flawed human being and do not profess to be anything else, yet Stella has always focused on anything but people's flaws, which is a big part of who she is.

The office opened in October 1987 and Stella started in June 1999, though I don't remember a year without her. Not only has she served as diplomatic envoy to a good portion of the more than fifty thousand patients who've come through our doors, but I've always considered her the keeper of the flame. No request is too big or too small. And I don't know how it started, but she has always taken it upon herself to open the door for me when I leave. No matter where she is or where I am in the office, somehow she zeroes in on the fact that I'm getting ready to go—her hand on the door handle before mine is. I've spent as much time as I could in my professional life trying to care for others, now leading me deeper into research and clinical trials, but the way she cares for me, my patients, and my practice overall cannot be defined by time or a particular action. It's simply who she is. In our mutual admiration society, however, she thinks that's who I am, so here are some of her recollections.

Stella in Her Words (Turkeys 'R Us)

"A lot of Dr. Haber's patients struggle to put food on the table. A few months after I started, he gave away turkeys for Thanksgiving, something he did for five or six years. These were actually huge frozen turkeys which sat in ice chests in the office. We had a list of people we knew would need them and we'd call them to come pick them up."

She recalls it was somewhat of a challenge because it was done the day before the holiday, and the turkey was frozen, so there was the question of whether or not it would defrost in time for families to actually eat it in time. Stella figured out a gift card would be more practical as people could use it to purchase the bird, the sides, and anything they might need to make their holiday special. Accordingly, the turkey endowment turned into gift card largesse.

"Sometimes we gave out a Christmas gift card," Stella also recalls, *"or even a birthday gift card for a cake or gift or meal in a restaurant. If a patient appointment happened to fall on or near a birthday and the patient mentioned it, the doctor would send one of us scurrying out to buy a present*

or a cake before they left. He'd have us ask the patient what he or she really wanted that day. We're talking about a very generous man.

"Many times during an exam, it came up that the patient didn't have insurance coverage for the prescription or the ability to afford it at all. Dr. Haber would call the pharmacy and have it charged to his account. There were other times a patient revealed they hadn't eaten in a couple of days, whereupon the doctor would send one of us across the street to buy hamburgers. It wasn't unusual for cash to be given to patients who couldn't buy food for their families or keep the lights on. For employees, gifts included large Christmas bonuses, spa gift cards, and other goodies as well.

"There are some here who are third generation Haber patients. He doesn't just treat the illness. He's concerned about their whole well-being. He always asks, 'Who do you live with? Who cooks for you? Who picks up your meds from the pharmacy? Do your kids come visit and bring your grandchildren? Have your daughter call me this afternoon because I want to talk with her about this.'"

"Famous for his forehead kissing and bear hugs which he considers an important component of healing and health maintenance, neither patients nor employees escape his feel good, endorphin-producing actions.

"One day I was home with bronchitis," Stella recalled. "Dr. Haber called to ask how I was feeling, and I told him I was feeling kind of weak. Next thing I knew he'd asked his housekeeper to prepare some soup for me. He's always considered his employees his extended family. How many doctors do that?

"For a long time Dr. Haber routinely made house calls. Some patients could not afford stretcher transportation, being bed bound. Consequently,

an adult child may not have been able to get their parent into a car, so the doctor would travel to the house. He's got a big, big heart. He constantly asks us how we are and if there are any office or other issues we may be having that he can help us with. It's an honor to work for him. I dread the day he retires because it will be a big loss for Laredo. There are a lot of new doctors coming up in the world, but there is only one Milton Haber."

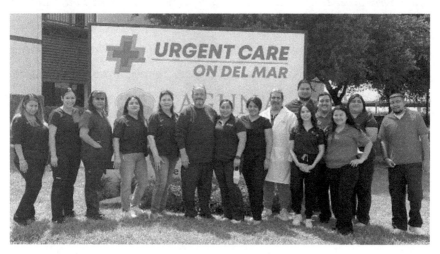

My staff with Stella Alvarez standing to the left with me in the center

Though Stella's memory is prodigious, and full of goodness, I do recall a thing or two from the early days of my practice when I was not all that pleasant a human being to deal with. I think Stella must have come aboard after a lot of the *tsuris*—a Yiddish word for turmoil—subsided, after I had mellowed somewhat, because while I always made patient and staff care a priority, it could be challenging to be around me. Okay, maybe sometimes it still is.

But before I explain all that, it's important to note practicing medicine was a learning curve for me. Just as it had taken me an hour to insert my first Swan Ganz catheter back in West Virginia, taking a patient history in my Laredo office took me the same amount of time. I soon discovered this would need to change if I wanted my practice to accommodate more than a handful of patients in a given month! I knew how to diagnose and treat, but running a medical practice like a well-oiled machine isn't something they teach you in medical school.

In my first year I was nervous. This wasn't so much about how to practice good medicine, as I was confident I was equipped to do that. But I had anxiety about building my practice, doing everything the right way in the process. I gained weight, becoming a compulsive eater, or in today's terms it'd be said, I was "eating my feelings." All true. Always in the back of my mind was that my father sold furniture to everyone, including a bunch of ninety-year-olds who probably didn't need it. He could sell, and I wanted to be able to sell as well because after all, I was in the position of saving lives, wasn't I? The only difference was the commodity I wanted to sell was me, not a lacquered coffee table. I wanted to sell myself to gain people's trust. I wanted Laredo to be assured I was doing something good for them, for their and their families' futures. I had something to prove to myself and everyone, at least that's the way I saw it.

I didn't take a day off, working fifteen- or sixteen-hour days, seven days a week for at least five years. The irony is as much as I never wanted to repeat my father's mistakes in rarely being around for his family, I was doing the exact same thing. My daughter Mariellen was born six years after her brother. I now had a wife and two small children and felt I was a very poor father because I was never around. My sole focus was medicine, and doing everything with great precision, but I knew I wasn't perfect and had to keep driving at it. Over the years, fortunately for myself and those around me, I have come to realize perfection in this life is unattainable. Yet I still strive to achieve it, though hopefully with more grace, compassion, and understanding.

In those days life was a constant struggle. As the saying goes, I was my own worst enemy. I was moody at times and undeniably aggressive in building my practice. In fact I can admit I was often a son-of-a-bitch though made it a point to always be polite to patients. In retrospect, the level of ambition I had comes with a kind of tunnel vision, and the first few years were a big test for me as a physician. Just as with the ECFMG referenced in chapter 3 so I could practice medicine in the US, I absolutely had to pass, and somehow it worked out. However now in my late sixties as I reflect back on the process, I don't quite know when or how a lot of things happened. I'm just grateful they did.

It all fell into place, perhaps part of the life script to which I keep referring. Who knows! At the risk of pontificating, or sounding as though I carry a rod and staff (Psalm 23), misrepresenting myself as some kind of holy person, that's not the point I'm trying to make. What I do know is that I kept working hard, increasingly tuning into my mistakes and the actions that led me there. So I believe not only did I pass the test of the first few years, but in time I became a less insistent, frenetic, impatient human being. There are days now where I slip back into my old ways, which probably won't ever go away completely, but at least I have an awareness about my behavior. If I can call up some measure of humility and admit it to myself, this allows me to make course corrections.

As a doctor I have always been cognizant of the fragility of life. Surviving the coronavirus, I'm acutely aware that our time on this earth is limited and if I fall off the good behavior wagon these days, it's only because I'm driving myself hard to provide my community with a legacy. I don't care about things like naming my research facility after me, the way many legacies are structured, which is why it's called Laguna Clinical Research Associates (for the street it's on). Name fame is not important to me. The goal is to be sure it is fully operational and sustainable, staffed by Laredo's finest medical personnel, making significant inroads into providing people opportunities to participate in clinical trials that previously were not available in Laredo. These opportunities very well may improve and save lives. It's also no small measure of satisfaction to me that people who participate in clinical trials are paid, so I know residents of my underserved community can have the option to supplement their incomes when appropriate.

The coronavirus and its implied comorbidities will ensure the longevity of many clinical trials as drugs and next generation drugs are developed to combat them. In addition to that, it is my hope and desire that Laguna will continue to participate in drug trials for other diseases, such as the lung cancer that took my mother, which has been defeating us for what seems like since time immemorial.

Rosa's Breath

How many of us think about our parents when they were children? I sometimes do, and this was especially common for me during the years I spent studying medicine in my mother's native country. Each time I traveled through big cities and into the countryside with my med school baseball team I thought of her some more, envisioning the joy she felt the day her family first saw Veracruz. When she was diagnosed with lung cancer at age sixty-four, and I'd missed identifying the symptoms for months, the realization plagued me for years to the point there were days I didn't think I'd survive. I'm a doctor, for God's sake. No one can know that kind of pain, and I kept it inside for decades, certain I was at fault, telling almost no one. I believed my mother, who loved me more than her own life, ultimately lost hers because of a fault in me. That belief in itself is like a cancer, dark and pernicious, releasing all kinds of mental and emotional toxins into the body that can eat away at your soul.

In 2013 some Catholic friends convinced me to accompany them to an ACTS Retreat, ACTS an acronym for adoration; community; theology; and service. In hindsight it must have taken some persuading because I am not of the Catholic faith and though I am Jewish, I am moderately so, practicing almost nothing. I came to learn, however, that the three-day lay retreat is more a kind of fellowship and catharsis than strict religious experience, where people are empowered to live fully. With that, I did find out I was the first Jew to participate in a Laredo ACTS Retreat.

The retreat had a significant purpose for me, making me understand that God accepted me not because I was in any way pure or perfect but because of my imperfections. By the end of the three days, and though I'd not raised the issue of the guilt I was carrying around, I did come to allow God's acceptance of me. In short I let Him in.

Four years later, after attending additional retreats, I was called upon to be a team member or facilitator. Veronica Procasky, who entered my life in 2013 and who factors enormously in it—someone I will fully introduce in the next chapter—helped me prepare a PowerPoint presentation. The theme was the John Lennon song *Imagine.* In that presentation I finally told the story of my mother's cancer, my years of keeping the intense guilt and grief to myself, and how being a part of ACTS changed all that for me. It's not an overstatement for me to say ACTS Retreats gave me my life back. I have to say when my presentation was over I felt an overwhelming sense of relief—relief like I'd never experienced before in all my life. In the days and weeks that followed, people would see me making rounds or out and about and ask what happened. I knew I was different: lighter. Veronica used the word glowing to describe me. If that's so, as the song says, imagine. Just imagine what would happen if we all came to a place of letting in acceptance—God's acceptance.

If it sounds as though I'm proselytizing, that's not my intention. What I want for everyone is what I have, though it has taken me years to get here. If I can save a little time for even one person, that's everything to me. That and making Laguna Clinical Research Associates a source of pride and national recognition for my community for at least the next hundred years. That's not a lot to ask!

6

In the Zone

"I long to accomplish a great and noble task, but it is my chief duty to accomplish small tasks as if they were great and noble."-Helen Keller

If you believe in a life script, in forming Laguna Clinical Research Associates the right people appeared when they were supposed to. Laguna would not have been established and growing the way it is without those key players. The longer I live, the more I understand that chance encounters and sudden events are part of a larger plan.

I've said a number of times I had a sense there was something missing in my life. I'd achieved so much but somewhere there was a lack. I was grateful for the kind of work I did, and that I could help people when they needed it, but over the years a voice in the background got louder and louder until I could no longer ignore it. I've heard this said by people who have made sweeping changes in their lives—maybe a car accident or serious illness reminded them just how short life is, sending them careening in another direction. While I certainly didn't want to rely on a trauma like that to precipitate change, nevertheless I felt my destiny could be elsewhere. Yes, I'd survived COVID-19, agonizing in itself and something I'll explore in more detail in the next chapter, though this itch for something else started years ahead of that. But the fact is I would not have been ready for my current journey earlier in my career. Thus the ancient script goes, "when the student is ready the teacher will appear." Some of those people who fit the teacher role in my life, opening my new life chapter and satisfying that deep professional yearning for a greater contribution to medicine, are Veronica Procasky and Chad Moore, co-founder of Elligo Health Research. I also want to tell you about Dr. Eduardo Miranda, a respected, honest, and ethical to a fault Laredo oncologist. He sets the bar quite high and is a good friend with whom I became involved in opening Laguna, but who was blindsided by unforeseen issues with the FDA. First, Veronica.

Veronica in Her Words

"In 2013 I was new to Specialty Hospital, working in compliance. My husband's job had brought us from the Midwest to New York, then by way of Houston to Laredo. Though Dr. Haber is an internist, who I met at Specialty Hospital, he is also considered a geriatrician because so many of his patients are elderly. One day during my incubation period there was a question about criteria for changing out Foley catheters from the various patients that came in to the hospital from long term care facilities or were transferred from another hospital. Apparently Dr. Haber had a reputation for not wanting input about things like this for his patients. He educated himself and implemented new standards based on his own medical expertise which is second to none. He has a reputation for being a strong advocate for his patients in all things, and to question him questions his character. When presented with suggestions from administrators, he listens, raises a fuss, and then processes what changes might need to be made, but not without a fight—the same fight he uses to bring the best care and services to his patients. Dr. Maurice Click who has known him for more than twenty years said the following: 'One thing is for sure. Dr. Haber may seem tough on the staff, hard on the administration, but it is all for his patients, and he will go to bat for them and their families.' He told me Dr. Haber's father was a big-time furniture store owner at one time in South Texas and that

he could be like him, all business when getting things done for his patients, just like his father did for his customers, but that he had the softness of his mother when interacting with patients themselves and their families. Dr. Click knew I had just arrived in Laredo and needed some guidance in addressing Dr. Haber's patients with him. He finished by giving me a stone cold gaze, saying, 'Don't mess with Haber's patients; just be good to the families and the patients and you'll be fine.'

"For the other doctors, we'd just assess patients to make helpful changes and suggestions and then get it done. Much to my dismay, I was somehow selected as the point person to educate Dr. Haber on the new CDC standards for Foley catheters. The corporate office wanted all doctors educated in this respect, but I was assigned to only one doctor for this task, the other case managers overseeing the other fifty. Staff more or less wished me good luck in talking to him. I approached him and he took a look at me, demanding to know who I was and where I was from.

"'Well…I'm Veronica, from the North," I smiled, or tried to. He could be just a little intimidating. He kept the line of questioning going, asking what I was doing in Laredo, where my husband was from, when we had arrived, and how long we'd be staying. I was confused and as he took charge of every word that came out of my mouth, it somehow did not seem the right time to talk about Foley catheters. Later I was at the administrative offices when I heard screaming and yelling in the hallway. I asked someone if they knew what was going on, not sure I wanted to look, and was told it was Dr. Haber. Listening more intently, I heard something about the computer system and ventured out. He was on a tirade about the administration office not using Cerner, state of the art software the hospital already used that related to medical records. The poor employee on the other end was catching heck. He wasn't letting up. I watched people come out of their offices to see what the commotion was about. When they saw who it was, they knowingly

shook their heads and filtered back to their desks. The director of case management came out and reassured him they'd get Cerner. His anxiety subsided and on his way out of the office, he grabbed a Martha Washington Celebration pictorial book.

"The Martha Washington Celebration is huge in Laredo. At a big coming out ceremony held once a year, young ladies are presented at a ball. The ceremony pictures, with the young ladies and their escorts and families, are published every year in a hardcover book in which local businesses pay for advertising. The book is then distributed to businesses throughout the city. A copy of it usually sits in every reception area throughout Laredo, and Dr. Haber's daughter happened to be in this one, along with his wife and son. He followed me and the case manager director into our office space, flipping through the book, telling me all about his children who he adores, Mariellen who was presented at the time, and his son Paul, whose free spirit reminds him of himself. I learned his wife Rita, a nurse practitioner, was a former Rockette NYC. It was nice that he wanted to show me all this, but a bit of a roller coaster ride for me that day—my introduction to Dr. Haber.

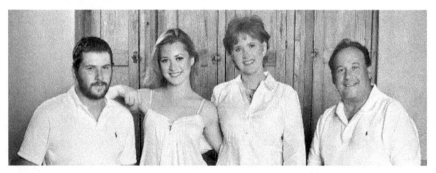

My family from left to right: Paul Haber, Mariellen Haber, Rita Haber, and me, Milton Haber, M.D. (Picture from Martha Washington Celebration Photos 2012)

"Shortly thereafter I decided I was interested in case management, more hands-on than compliance, and was assigned to him. It was no picnic. I'd walk down the hall and he'd act as though he didn't see me. Questioning colleagues about this behavior, I'd get the same refrain: 'You have your plan of care and he has his.' Weeks passed like this and one day he actually spoke to me in the hallway.

"'You're a nurse,' Dr. Haber said to me, adding someone had just informed him. I said yes, bracing myself, unsure of what was coming. 'I thought you were just an attorney,' he responded, i.e. a non-clinical attorney assigned to evaluate his documentation processes.

"Translation: for a long time he was under the impression I was there to monitor him, in an official capacity, something he might have construed as stalking and certainly nothing he would have appreciated! I guess that wasn't far from the truth, though now, working together as we do at Laguna, I am always looking out for him."

Veronica remembers our first few meetings as being less than auspicious, but I've never denied I can be difficult. She is a registered nurse who graduated from law school in 2011. She is the key and cornerstone to this phase of my life where I'm expanding into research and clinical trials. Utilizing her medical and legal expertise, she's helping me open congruent urgent care centers to care for my clinical trials participants who may have side effects from various medications or vaccines, and for others in the community who need healing as well. These include the colleague mentioned earlier, oncologist Dr. Eduardo Miranda, who was involved with me in our foray into clinical trials. In fact he was there first, his work inspiring me to do it. And though he needed healing, Dr. Miranda's needs were of a different kind and on a larger scale. It was a legal issue with the FDA that had the potential to derail him. I arranged a meeting between Veronica and my friend Eduardo. Fortunately they both liked sushi.

About Dr. Miranda

Between 2007 and 2009, years before supply chain regulation was marked by 2013's passage of Obama Administration-sponsored US Drug Quality and Security Act, a drug shortage of the anti-nausea medication Kytril (generic: Granisetron) existed. An extremely effective drug to combat the side effects of cancer treatment, Dr. Miranda was suddenly unable to obtain it. An office administrator came across a faxed advertisement (no longer legal though they were at the time) for a US pharmacy that purportedly stocked it. Unbeknownst to the hundreds of doctors around the country who availed themselves of Kytril from this venue and were eventually implicated by the FDA, the drug was being fraudulently funneled to a warehouse in the US from Canada.

One of only two oncologists in Laredo, someone I and others on the board of Doctor's Hospital hired away from Phoenix in 1998-99, Dr. Miranda's practice was massive. Accordingly he required a robust inventory of Kytril to meet patient demand. What's important to note about Dr. Miranda is in all the years he'd been practicing in Laredo, if a patient couldn't pay, he never denied them care or medication and never sent an account to collection. His patients' health was and continues to be his priority, and for the majority of them, Kytril was the most effective anti-nausea drug he could prescribe. The prices from the advertised pharmacy also happened to be lower than they were when the drug was in ready supply in other places, as were a few other medications he ended up ordering from this supplier as he'd now had success with them. All of this gave the FDA, FBI, and DEA more ammunition to raid his office in 2009 and eventually end up prosecuting him.

To make matters worse, Dr. Miranda initially hired a local attorney who wrongly advised him to plead guilty instead of fighting the misdemeanor charge, just to get it over with. That pivotal mistake has had a domino effect on his career. The rumor mill turned and he falsely-labeled for a felony charge which was got the ear of Texas Medical Board. Where his practice was concerned, the ill-advised decision to plead guilty also curtailed his ability to participate in federal funding programs such as Medicare and Medicaid until 2026, backfiring on the patients whose lives he cared about more than anything.

Though she'd only just passed the bar, I asked Veronica to work with him to extricate him from this mess—to clear his good name. She felt it would be excellent training ground for private practice one day which was her goal. Still employed by Specialty Hospital, she'd leave work at the end of the day to spend a few hours at Dr. Miranda's office reviewing hundreds of documents, devising a fighting strategy to redeem his privileges and reputation. She was also there on weekends, subordinating time with her husband and son to the cause. At one point she even wrote a letter to the President of the United States requesting a pardon—an issue that is still pending in the Presidential Pardon Office. Her pro bono work continued for three years, followed by an offer to become his official general counsel, which she accepted for a while. To date everything but the federal charge and an ongoing exclusion/waiver with Centers for Medicare and Medicaid Services (CMS) has been dismissed with the pardon still pending. The fact is following the 2009 raid, the misdemeanor simply went on the federal docket for a few years with absolutely no action taken. Charges were not pressed right away. In 2013, when he ventured into research and clinical trials becoming more prominent in the local medical community, and also somewhat nationally, the federal government decided to pull the trigger. The statute of limitations was set to expire the following year but the feds decided to move. On advice from his attorney at the time he pled guilty; his professional life began to unravel.

In addition to being my good friend and esteemed colleague, Dr. Miranda's experience in research and clinical trials was exemplary. I wanted in. I wanted to be a part of something of this magnitude with the potential to change people's lives. At first, my interest had been in opening a group of urgent care centers to better serve marginalized residents of Laredo and surrounding areas, but when I understood the power of clinical trials, I knew they could go hand in hand. Rather than running trials out of my office, and Dr. Miranda out of his as he'd been doing, in 2018 Veronica helped us form Laguna Clinical Research Associates. Veronica suggested we adopt a model from MD Anderson Cancer Center that uses both clinical trials and urgent care centers and refined it, tailoring it to our vision. In time the goal is to have ten to twenty small town clinical trials and urgent care centers throughout the Southwest. Timing was excellent for our debut as a little more than a year later, following the studies we got from Bristol Meyers and Novartis, the coronavirus hit and we won a contract from Moderna to conduct its vaccine trials in South Texas.

Dr. Miranda In His Words

"*When I came to Laredo in 1999, there were one hundred seventy-seven thousand residents. It was the second fastest growing city in the country,* behind Las Vegas. With only one oncologist and no university hospital with its implied support, the need for another doctor was great. Patients were going out of town to the closest oncology facility, one hundred sixty miles away.

"In my experience, people whose thinking aligns with another tend to form a friendship. Dr. Haber and I saw things the same way and our professional relationship and friendship grew from the beginning. When I first arrived in Laredo, the family of a middle-aged patient diagnosed with ovarian cancer that had spread to the lungs and abdomen pushed for her to be transferred to San Antonio or Houston. But we'd been developing a successful cancer treatment program in Laredo. Together Dr. Haber and I told the patient and her family she could deteriorate on the trip and we needed to keep her in Laredo—we had the capability to treat her right here. He was very insistent, as he can be. We finally prevailed and many years later she's still alive. Dr. Haber has great confidence in how we do things which he's had ever since I've known him. Patient care and doing things better are what matter most to him. The same for Laguna Clinical Research Associates, which is an alliance of doctors with the same ideals. In fact, and because Dr. Haber and Veronica crusaded throughout Laredo for Moderna vaccine trial participants, I was one of the first to sign up!

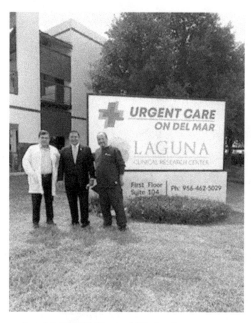

Eduardo Miranda, M.D. (left) and U.S. Congressman Henry Cuellar (center) with me (right) in front of the Laguna Research Center

"I've always seen great energy in Dr. Haber. He's always making plans. Build this; expand that; do something big! And it's not just talk. One success motivates him to go for more: he wants to do a lot of great things. I'm a realist and he's more optimistic than I am—it's good to be around someone like that. He's also at the age when many of us are slowing down, making plans for retirement, but he's making plans for the next project. We love what we do; it motivates us. But he goes beyond that."

Moving Forward

Through Veronica's diligence we found and partnered with Elligo Health Research, a technology-enabled services company that makes it possible for clinical research facilities like ours to conduct clinical trials. Laguna is different than a lot of facilities tied to large hospitals or universities. We are new and small and needed all the help we could get. It proved to be a good working relationship and we knew we could rely on them to help us grow. We came to a point where Veronica and I realized that Dr. Miranda's FDA issue would present a liability to future growth of Laguna with Elligo. Though Dr. Miranda willingly stepped aside, the situation was like a blow to my soul. Veronica and I knew his standard of ethics and altruism far exceeded anything, and that through no fault of his own he'd been blindsided. But given the number and caliber of drug studies Elligo had been delivering to us, and would continue to, there was no question we needed them more than him, harsh as it sounds. Sometimes business is a beast with which you have to grapple. This was something Dr. Miranda understood though there are days and weeks I question just how much more he can bear—how much any one of us should have to take. Somehow, though stripped of many of the resources he needs to fully support his patients, he keeps his practice going. Patients respect and support him, knowing what's in his heart, exactly who he is, and that he'll get to the other side of this. He was very well liked by Elligo and his hard work appreciated, but all that had transpired which played out on a local and federal stage would likely prevent Elligo from moving forward with us to the extent that we needed to expand. I keep positive thoughts that all will be resolved and he will join us once again.

Chad Moore, Elligo co-founder, strategic advisor and former president, In His Words

"'I love you' is what Dr. Haber said at the end of our first telephone conversation. I wasn't exactly sure what I heard! But the next time we spoke, he did it again. As you get to know him, you understand that unlike many people in business where you're never sure what their real agenda is,

and you deal with a thick façade, his isn't thick. In fact there is no façade at all. He is so open and accessible every patient has his cell phone number.

"In 2016 my business partner John Potthoff and I founded Elligo which is from the Latin meaning to choose a few from many, precisely what we do in clinical research. It's actually correctly spelled with one 'l' but we had to add one as there's a bioscience company in Switzerland that spells it the other way.

"In the middle of 2015, John and I wanted to form a company together. We knewclinical research was inefficient and accessible only by those people who happen to be close to a participating facility. In addition, we heard stories about people who would have loved to participate in a research study, but they didn't know how to find out about them. John's barber learned he had cancer. Being the kind of person he is, John scoured the country, ultimately finding a clinical trial three hours away in Houston at MD Anderson for which the barber would qualify. It would involve numerous trips back and forth—every two or three weeks for several months for a half-day visit. He couldn't believe his luck, but when he told the barber, it was impossible. The barber said, 'If I'm not cutting hair, I'm not making money, and if I'm not making money, I'm not taking care of my family. It's too far; I just can't participate.' He ended up passing away. Who can say if participating in the study would have made a difference, but his loss had a huge impact on John and me.

"The impetus for us in designing Elligo was to bring clinical trials to the masses—to democratize it—to bring research opportunities to anyone that qualifies and would like to participate.. In the US and throughout the world, research is traditionally conducted only at discrete and unique locations such as MD Anderson and the Mayo Clinic. The FDA has said for years it needs to do more community research, so Elligo does two primary

things: (1) partner with healthcare systems and providers to make research available in areas where opportunities to conveniently participate in research is lacking and (2) design and conduct decentralized clinical trials—where patients participate largely from their homes using technology and receiving home visits from healthcare providers. Elligo has to be discerning in deciding where we go for the most successful outcomes. The Moderna vaccine study was part of a thirty thousand-participant study nationwide. It was Dr. Haber's connection with and vision for his community, his passion, confidence, and enthusiasm for research that convinced us Laguna could execute the trials. We knew we could count on his leadership and direction. He has been a top performer who has exceeded our expectations."

If You Build It...

It bears saying in this chapter just how hands on Veronica and I were in creating our research facility and first urgent care center: Urgent Care on Del Mar. As a teen I'd had that construction job where I hauled planks and hammered nails for Doctor's Hospital, where, astonishingly, I'd eventually have physician privileges. Veronica caught the building bug.

From Veronica

"Before we opened, I went shopping myself. I bought everything from the ground up, framing pictures and assembling furniture with my own hands, trying to be judicious and keep things on a shoestring.

"One day I put together a phlebotomy chair, 'humbly' telling a coworker I thought she would just love the color of the chair that I had so carefully selected for the clinic! She asked me who put it together as she'd seen it

delivered in a box a few days earlier. I excitedly told her I had done it myself. I laid everything out and put in all the screws with the intention of tightening them later. But it was still dark in the clinic as we didn't yet have electricity. I decided to push it out into the lobby where there was some light to show her the color and when I did, everything popped off. You want blood to come from a needle stick—not a chair collapse. Needless to say I relinquished some of my hands-on work at that point. But we were so committed to having this happen for the community, there's nothing we wouldn't do."

When COVID hit and we got the Moderna vaccine trials, I can't say enough times that I was beyond grateful. Now I would get to help my community in a very big way. But acquiring the study was only half the battle. Statistically, minorities including Blacks and Latinos are reluctant to participate in trials, and in some cases to take the vaccine in the first place, so what good would it do to have the study if we couldn't implement it?

Moderna asked us to target three hundred participants and not to limit it to patients of mine. That meant Veronica and I had to go out into the community essentially door to door. She did just that, walking up and down streets handing out flyers while getting me interviewed on TV news programs and in the newspapers, on radio, podcasts, social media, and more. We launched a campaign on par with someone running for office, except that the victor wouldn't be a single individual. It'd be hundreds of residents of the Laredo community. All benefitting. All winners.

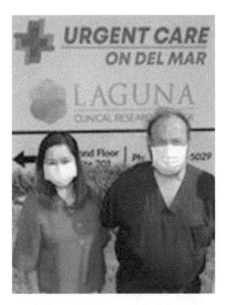

Maria Monette Regalado, M.D., my Sub-Investigator on the Moderna study, standing with me in front of Laguna Clinical Research Center

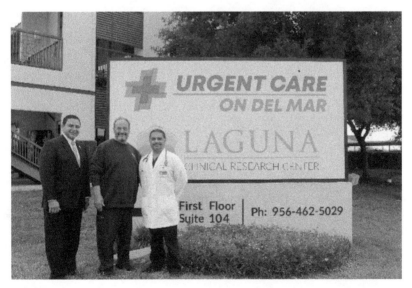

U.S. Congressman Henry Cuellar, who supported bringing Moderna's study to Laredo, with me (center) and Ron Meza (right), another one of my Sub-Investigators on the Moderna study

7

In the Lab

"Although the world is full of suffering, it is also full of overcoming it." -Helen Keller

Some people resist the idea of vaccines. In the age of soundbites, abbreviations, hashtags, and monikers, they are the so-called "anti-vaxxers." Opposition is a mindset that can arise with anything new or unknown, not just vaccines, and history tells us where vaccines are concerned this is not a new problem. In the early 1800s, people expressed sanitary, religious, and/or political opposition to being injected with part of a cowpox blister to protect them from smallpox. In the 1970s the DTP vaccine for diphtheria, tetanus, and pertussis was met with skepticism when it was linked to neurological disorders, though studies claimed the risk was very low. Autism-related issues surrounding the use of vaccines in general seem always to be part of the conversation.

Among some populations, general distrust of clinical trials and vaccines is fomented by the ill-conceived and unconscionable Tuskegee incident, officially "the Tuskegee Study of Untreated Syphilis in the Negro Male." This has never been forgotten or forgiven, nor should it be. Conducted from 1932 to 1972 by the US Public Health Service and Centers for Disease Control and Prevention, Black males were unwittingly subjected to what was called the natural study of untreated syphilis. This heinous act by the federal government, carried out with traditionally Black college Tuskegee University, tricked six hundred impoverished sharecroppers from Macon County, Alabama, into believing they were receiving free health care. Though never informed of the conditions they had, three hundred ninety-nine had latent syphilis while the remainder of the group did not.

Participants were told the study would last six months; it went on for forty years even after funding disappeared. Infected participants were never given penicillin though it had become widely available by 1947 and was the recommended method of treatment. There was never any intention of treating these men, and the study caused the death of one hundred twenty-eight of them either directly from syphilis or related complications. This travesty of government, medicine, and conscience has left an indelible stain on the nation and particularly on the Black population. For thousands of those whose families suffered and others who simply remember, or have studied it, it's no mystery there is so much distrust. It's not hard to understand why they may be reluctant to participate in anything remotely redolent of that time.

By association, and though it is growing by leaps and bounds, the Hispanic population also tends to identify with minorities mistreated in clinical research, so there is that hurdle for us to overcome. And, of course today there is increasing widespread mistrust of the US government, though hopefully with the kinds of safeguards, checks, and balances medicine has in place today, Tuskegee could never again happen.

Where the coronavirus vaccine is concerned, in this chapter I'm going to break it all down. My apologies in advance for anything too technical. My intention is to provide complete and comprehensive information as succinctly as possible—information that allays people's fears and reservations.

Manufacturing Greatness—Not Opposition

First, it's important to understand ribonucleic acid, or RNA, and the role it plays in the vaccine. If the term takes you back to long nights studying for a dreaded biology exam, you may want to rethink that part of your education and the invaluable information you gained from it. Forms of RNA include transfer RNA (tRNA), ribosomal RNA (rRNA), and messenger RNA (mRNA). So why is this important here? It's the messenger RNA I'm going to focus on right now because it makes the coronavirus vaccine as effective as it is. In fact largely because of it, there is every reason to take the vaccine.

Some of us are under the impression the vaccine is a live virus, hence the reason for avoiding it. It is not. The vaccine cannot give you COVID-19. The vaccine creates an antigen which antibodies (T cells—which participate in the immune response) recognize as foreign, attacking what's called the M spike protein it creates. Simply put the result is it doesn't allow the virus to enter the cell, which is how people are protected. Further, as second generation vaccines are being developed, they're even better by being more specific to the M spike proteins than the first generation. The vaccine is comprised of mRNA with a lipid particle to improve penetration, preserve it, and slow down elimination so it can be as fully absorbed as possible.

A little deeper into the weeds, mRNA for vaccines has been studied for twenty years or more. Until the use of mRNA, vaccines were at risk for not being fully absorbed by the body. Now considered mainstream, mRNA with the addition of a lipid particle has opened the door to more effective outcomes in combating the Zika virus, rabies, HIV, and other deadly diseases. Again, I realize this is a lot of technical information, and it was a lot to throw at the people we were trying to enroll in the COVID clinical trials. But this is important and as the saying goes knowledge is power, and making decisions without correct and complete knowledge can lead to wrong decisions—such as rejecting the vaccine. While it may not be 100 percent effective in all who receive it, it's as close as it can be now and even if you contract COVID-19 down the road, the science data shows that its effects are mitigated by availing yourself the vaccine. Why? You're developing neutralizing antibodies that can last up to a year. Sure, a booster may become necessary. But with prudent use of masks and social distancing for the time being, forecasters say in a year or so the coronavirus will largely be in the rear view mirror, as was smallpox, DTP, polio, and other viruses. What's more, as mentioned, with each new generation of the vaccine its efficacy and protection are expected to improve, which will provide an even better reason to receive it at the time it's offered. Though I sometimes feel we shouldn't have to sell the idea the way we do, I've taken on that responsibility and not a day passes when Veronica and I don't try and figure out a better way to help people by getting the message out. So here are a few things to think about when considering the vaccine:

Got a job to maintain?
Children who depend on you?
A spouse who loves you?
Aging parents who need you?

In short, what have we got to lose? Possibly everyone and everything if we don't get the vaccine when we can.

At this time, the US government is undertaking public initiatives including community engagement to encourage people to get the vaccine. On December 27, 2020, the President signed into law the *FY 2021 Coronavirus Response and Relief Supplemental Appropriations Act of 2021.* Included is the following:

Increase vaccine confidence through education, outreach, and partnerships • Enhance/amplify messaging (including through translation) to promote COVID-19 vaccination, especially among underserved populations (see also CLAS Standards - Think Cultural Health (hhs. gov) • Fund local education campaigns and approaches to adapting CDC materials to community audiences, including a focus on racial and ethnic minority groups • Share educational, outreach and marketing approaches and materials with CDC and others engaged in similar activities to allow for national dissemination. Recipients are reminded to be cognizant of the statutory and policy requirements for acknowledging HHS/CDC funding when issuing statements, press releases, publications, requests for proposal, bid solicitations and other documents in accordance with CDC General Terms and Conditions for Non-research Awards - Acknowledgement of Federal Funding in your base award. • Address vaccine education efforts to include addressing possible vaccine misinformation and increase vaccine confidence and vaccine uptake, including with racial and ethnic minority groups • Fund local health department contracts to promote COVID-19 and other vaccinations to increase vaccine confidence in racial and ethnic minority groups and to increase accessibility for people with disabilities.

Develop and implement community engagement strategies to promote COVID-19 vaccination efforts • Support broad education efforts that explain to the public options for how/where/when they can get COVID-19 vaccine in their communities • Fund partnerships for community engagement to identify trusted voices that represent the diversity of affected communities to promote vaccination and have bidirectional conversations in communities with vaccine hesitancy. These partnerships need to reflect the diversity of the jurisdiction's population. • Implement a rapid community assessment guide to diagnose potential barriers and identify solutions to low vaccine uptake or vaccine confidence in specific communities. • Fund community-based organizations and build local partnerships or coalitions to allow for coordinated activities across community organizations working to promote vaccine confidence. Examples of community-based organizations include social service agencies, nonprofit organizations, and formal and informal community groups, like neighborhood groups or recreational or special-interest clubs.

Support high vaccination uptake in tribal nations • As applicable, provide funding to support Tribal Health Programs and Urban Indian Organizations (e.g., for supplies, educational/communication materials, storage and handling equipment). Any funding provided to Tribal Health Programs and Urban Indian Organizations should complement efforts supported through the Indian Health Service. • Collaborate with Tribal organizations to develop culturally appropriate materials for their specific American Indian/Alaska Native (AI/AN) populations, as appropriate. • Partners to consider funding include, but are not limited to: √ Tribal Health Programs and Urban Indian Organizations √ Tribal Epidemiology Centers (TECs) √ Area Indian Health Boards NCIRD COVID-19 Supplemental Funding Guidance – January 2021 8 Revised 1/13/2021 √ Tribal WIC programs √ Tribal daycares √ Association of American Indian Physicians (AAIP) local affiliates √ National Association of Indian Nurses of America (NAINA) local affiliates √ Tribal & Urban Indian Health Immunization Coalition √ Alaskan Native Tribal Health Consortium (ANTHC).

Distrust and barriers do not exist solely in this country. Many people throughout the world don't trust science, something I've been aware of through thirty-four years in private practice. Like it or not, the pandemic has put science smack in the middle of our living rooms, bedrooms, and more, and for the first time I feel the tide turning. How we approach the virus is determining that change. The playing out of the pandemic took place largely in a politically-charged environment, amplified by the media, which only served to exacerbate people's mistrust of the process. Yet it's a wise and strategic use of media, including social media as Veronica and I did to inform the people of Laredo of the opportunity to participate in the Moderna COVID-19 trials—to educate people about the merits of the vaccine. Unfortunately many doctors, scientists, and the like are not all that skilled at employing social media, but that will need to change with the unfortunate projection of other pandemics in the future.

With the speed at which the big drug companies whisked the vaccine to market, educational information was lacking about the steps it takes to get it safely out there to reassure the general public. Consequently, people were left to question the process, further compounding the issue of whether or not to take the vaccine. In a sense, though, the activity around developing, releasing, and marketing the COVID-19 vaccine has thrust open the door to a more efficient and expedited process in the development of other vaccines. This will become essential to our survival in the immediate and long-term future, with emerging variants and the threat of other pandemics on the horizon. But again—and if you'll allow me to reach back and use one of my favorite baseball terms—the fact-based information machine is going to have to step up to the plate in ways it never has before. Without it, vaccines will be ineffective only because people will have reservations about taking them.

Long Haulers and Comorbidities

It's undeniable that more than a year into the pandemic, the impact on those affected has varied tremendously. Post-COVID, some patients appear to have no health repercussions while others experience varying degrees of fatigue, ongoing shortness of breath, brain fog or confusion, loss of smell or taste, etc. The lungs of virus sufferers generally become scarred, some requiring ventilators and in others damaged enough to kill them no matter what measures are taken. Yet we have no way of knowing about clinical manifestations five or ten years from now. Can the virus cause cancer, for example? This is something that interests me and I hope that down the road Laguna Clinical Research Associates can explore this possibility. Long after we recover, the coronavirus has the potential to impact our hearts, gastrointestinal tracts, kidneys, bones, skin, and brains, including causing neurological issues. And what about post-COVID pediatric complications? Some patients today commonly report depression that lingers, even becoming chronic, many months after they are pronounced virus-free. In the next ten years I wouldn't be surprised if we saw more disability claims than ever before in the history of this country. Accordingly, our post-COVID economy will need to be restructured to accommodate them.

Do You Know Me?

It's old news that historically medical schools have not taught classes in doctor-patient relationships. I'm not talking about the privacy issue, but rather how crucial it is that knowing everything about the patient—daily habits; personal and environmental challenges; nutrition concerns; family involvement; life changes—as I've tried to do for more than three decades can mean the difference between a patient living or dying. In chapter 5, my office receptionist Stella Alvarez talked about my tendency to "interview"—or maybe cross examine is more accurate—my patients each time I see them, no matter how long they've been a part of my practice, to determine if there is anything in their lives that needs to be addressed. If I prescribe medication, can they afford it? Can they read the label? Can they physically get to the store to obtain it? If not, can a family member or friend pick it up and if they live alone, monitor how they're doing on it? Do they need home health visits? Again, as a rule they don't teach this kind of investigative medicine in med school, though you'd have thought it would have changed since the '80s when I was grinding my way through. It has not. There are programs here and there that insert a class into the curriculum, but this aspect of medicine is largely overlooked even today. In fact, in today's corporate and team approaches to medicine, doctors rely more on other doctors, resulting in less personal connection to the patient. Bringing it into the context of this chapter, that relationship can make a difference in a reluctant patient taking the vaccine or not. It's precisely this kind of support that can overcome any obstacles, thereby impacting who lives or dies.

When I got COVID-19 and ended up spending nearly a week in the intensive care unit, which I will talk about in the next chapter, the doctors who made a real effort to connect with me made a difference. Aside from labs and vitals, talking and listening is so important. You hear stories from time to time about doctors who see patients but really don't *see* them, and could be phoning it in from Uruguay or the moon.

There were times I pretty much hovered between life and death and needed more than a cold stethoscope on my chest. I needed a warm, reassuring hand on my shoulder. In medicine, as in life, I've always believed you have to show some concern, some intention, some empathy. You have to make a connection.

8

In the Light

"Life is slippery. Here, take my hand." – H. Jackson Browne, Jr.

If you have children and they're away at school, you know the feeling when they come home. You can't wait and you can't get enough of them. I'd been a workaholic for the first long years of my son and daughter's lives and though I'm still undeniably driven about my work, I hope I'm there more for them now. Sometimes I can't believe the kind, generous, accomplished young adults they've become, mostly because of my wife Rita. But inasmuch as my daughter Mariellen is in medical school, following in the footsteps of her proud dad, I probably didn't make too many mistakes there.

In early December, 2020, Mariellen came home from medical school in Arizona. COVID was raging and schools were operating if not fully, than partially, on a remote basis. We were also into the holiday season and Rita and I looked forward to spending time with her and our son Paul.

I was working from home over the weekend with telemedicine in full swing. On Saturday evening I really wasn't feeling too well, tired and maybe kind of warm. I didn't have a sore throat, though I did possibly have some semblance of a cough, but nothing other than that. Next morning I called Veronica and told her I wanted my daughter and her boyfriend screened for COVID. The idea had been on my mind just because of my line of work and as a parent we want to protect our children, adult or otherwise. Veronica recalls at the time we spoke what I thought was just a mild cough became more pronounced in the course of conversation. She asked me what was going on. Clearly in light of the virus, gone are the days when adults get sick and say it's nothing, or tough it out so as not to miss a day of work. Today, responsibly, the first sign of illness is the starting gun to stay home, take it easy, and get tested. But I'll be honest. At that point my thinking wasn't inclined toward actually having caught the virus myself.

From Veronica

"Mariellen had only just arrived the night before. If Dr. Haber had COVID, I knew it couldn't have been from her as it would have been too soon for any symptoms. I told him I was going into the office to update policies and procedures, something we do annually, and I called urgent care to let them know family members were coming in for testing. Before Dr. Haber and I hung up, I said 'let me know if you need any testing.' I don't think he took me seriously.

"Around 2 p.m. he called me, saying he really believed he needed to be tested. At first I thought he was kidding. He said he had a low grade fever and didn't want to get anybody sick so he'd stay in his car, whereupon I met him at urgent care parking lot. Dr. Haber's nurse practitioner, Marco Vela, came out to swab him with me trailing behind making sure Marco had all the necessary supplies in hand. In his customary manner (ahem!), Dr. Haber pulled his head to the side, telling Marco he wanted me to do it and he wanted it done gently, not like the swabbing that is done by Marco. Marco and I exchanged looks, sensing the fear in an otherwise invincible doctor. We did a rapid COVID antigen and antibody test which would

come back in fifteen minutes. In his inimitable style Dr. Haber wouldn't let me push the swab back far enough in the nose, Marco commenting he didn't think we got a good sample. He was right, as the rapid test came back negative. Looking at the results, intuiting the doctor's nervousness and the possibility the sample was not adequate, we decided we wanted a polymerase chain reaction test, or PCR, which would take up to a few days for results but is the definitive test for the virus. We took his vitals and a fever of 101 registered, so we went ahead and drew blood for a full lab workup. He's usually the one giving orders but now we were. In a show of bravado Dr. Haber started making light about coding and us intubating him—the complete opposite behavior of the way he cares for his patients as he takes these things so seriously. I knew it was a façade for the underlying fear he felt that if he were indeed sick, after his work on the clinical trials and months as a frontline worker, it would be hard for him to accept that the doctor was now the patient."

The next day I really didn't feel well. My labs showed I was dehydrated. I wanted to think it was the flu, which was always possible. I had a home health nurse come by my house to give me a liter of IV fluids, deciding to call my good friend and colleague in San Antonio, cardiologist Dr. Robert Schnitzler, to run this by him. He said he thought it was COVID and at 8:45 p.m., Veronica called and the PCR test had confirmed it. The home health nurse returned on Tuesday to administer more fluids. I was so fatigued and weak by that point I couldn't get out of bed. Because I'm a doctor I guess I was falling hard—struggling to believe I was not invincible and yes, okay, it was really happening to me. There was no getting around it. Dr. Schnitzler and I spoke again wherein he asked me if I wanted to go to San Antonio to see him. San Antonio is two and a half hours away and I thought I could handle it at home. Heck, I'm a doctor, and I had a home healthcare nurse coming in, checking my vitals and wrangling IV fluids.

That night, after the nurse had come and gone, I decided I just had to get out of bed. I was weak and a little disoriented. The IV tube pulled back and I went down, striking myself on an iron bedside table. The pain to the left chest wall was excruciating—of blackout caliber though I didn't quite lose consciousness. I was short of breath and cut my arm. The noise brought my wife and daughter flying into the room, flashing on my panicked dog licking me as I lay on the floor. They got me back into bed and I called Dr. Schnitzler to tell him what happened. My breathing was quite compromised as I relayed the situation; I was certain I fractured some ribs and worried if a lung had been punctured as a result.

"Get yourself to San Antonio," Dr. Schnitzler ordered. "Now."

My good friend Hector Medina owns BronzeStar Ambulance. Because of the pandemic he couldn't coerce any of his crew to come get me, so he cuirassed himself in a hazmat suit, looking every bit like the astronauts in *2001: A Space Odyssey*. Maybe more appropriately he looked like Dustin Hoffman in *Outbreak*—the 1995 film about containing the spread of a lethal virus. Interestingly, the film was based on Richard Preston's nonfiction bestseller *The Hot Zone* about origins and incidents of viral hemorrhagic fevers—nonfiction being the operative word here.

Just ahead of Hector's arrival, my wife and daughter helped me to the front steps where I sat holding a small baggie with a change of underwear. At that point I could barely move: walking was a Herculean effort and I was in too much pain from the broken ribs to lie down on a gurney. Hector put his arm around me and somehow got me into the ambulance, a magical feat on his part, where of course I still could not lie down so he had me sit on the side of the gurney. Though I tried to keep the pain to myself, it was the most torturous one hundred fifty miles I've ever ridden in my life. I thought back to the road trip and California vacation my family had spent together in 1962, ending up on horseback in Texas's Big Bend National Park, galloping at top speed over rocky terrain. If my body felt any pain from the wild ride back then, which it likely did, it was masked by an explosion of endorphins that marked one of the best days of my life. But today surely was not one of those. Every bump in the road or even a slight application of the brakes ricocheted through my body like a hail of bullets. Rita and Mariellen followed behind in the car, and I was incredibly grateful we were not together because I can't begin to imagine how much my pain would have upset them.

In San Antonio, Methodist Hospital was full so we diverted to Full Spectrum ER and Urgent Care, known as a stat hospital. It was close to Methodist and I'd be able to immediately transition to Methodist following Spectrum protocol. ER staff was waiting for me, per Dr. Schnitzler, though they were probably surprised when I walked in pretty much in Hector's arms as opposed to being wheeled in on a gurney. At this point my left leg was also hurting. What else! The emergency room doctor had to give me a whole gram of Dilaudid just so I could change positions enough to lie down for the CT scan. This would ascertain if my lungs, spleen, and/or diaphragm were ruptured as a result of the fall. Turns out they weren't. The ER doc said I didn't appear to have pneumonia but he was wrong, I clearly had pneumonia, soon determined by the pulmonologist.

I transferred to Methodist Hospital around 3:30 a.m., so depleted and in so much agony the nurses had to do everything. Two more milligrams of Dilaudid did something for the pain, but for all intents and purposes I was flaccid. I barely recall being started on oxygen, later awaking to find a cannula in my nose. There it was: doctor as patient. By way of another popular reference, there's a 1991 movie, *The Doctor*, starring William Hurt as a hotshot surgeon. Famously callous, abrasive, and entirely disconnected from his patients and also from his family, when diagnosed with cancer he has a reckoning from which he emerges transformed: the kind of human being he'd never have become had he not been brought to his knees. While clearly I was not rude to nor disconnected from my patients, in the days that followed I was about to experience a profound transformation as well.

Coming and Going

It's a fact of life that we come into this world alone and go out alone. There's nothing we can do about it. But in between, human beings are not wired to be solitary creatures. To my thinking, COVID-19 is the first disease of such mammoth proportion and duration where we've been separated from others. Fundamentally, it's a challenging enough predicament, but when you add in the extreme isolation when people are lying alone in hospital beds without the benefit of family support, it's nothing less than a formula for disaster.

In the week I spent in the ICU, due to COVID restrictions I saw no one except for nurses who came in every few hours and rounding doctors. I was very sick but not too sick to feel, especially loss like this—and it really is a form of loss. I'm not a good patient though I did my best to cooperate, actually finding myself counting down the time to the fleeting moments of human contact—even eye contact and brief conversation. Aside from what the virus was doing and the possibility of my getting even worse feeling like a chokehold sometimes, all the hours I was left alone took another kind of toll.

There's a story that circulated some years ago called "The Rescuing Hug." Twins were born, placed in separate incubators. In the first week of their lives, one was tinier, frail, and struggling, not expected to survive. A nurse fought against hospital rules and placed both babies in the same incubator. The healthier of the two placed her arm around her sister in an endearing embrace. The smaller baby's heart rate stabilized and her temperature rose to normal. The end of the story says "let us not forgot to embrace those whom we love." There are statistics that have been around for decades about babies in orphanages failing to thrive for the lack of human contact. This is nothing new, but when you experience it for the first time, even as an adult there is no disputing it.

The separation of families during the pandemic, with loved ones fighting for their lives and dying alone in hospitals, had been on my mind but never more than when I lay in that ICU bed. I've said before I tend to be an optimist by nature, to which my friend Dr. Miranda attested in chapter 6, but this was the hour of the ultimate test. When I could be moved to a chair by the window, I spent hours looking out, putting my face to the sun. A few times I actually sat there long enough to see it move across the sky and set at the end of the day. I saw planes taking off and feeling sorry for myself, wished I were on them—going anywhere—anywhere but here. I was keenly aware of the fragility of life, certainly of my own life at that point. Alone like that there was a lot of time to think. My predominant thoughts were that I wanted to be around people I cared about: Rita and my children. I thought about Stella, my friends, close colleagues like Veronica, Dr. Miranda and Chad, my vision for my research work, and others who really cared about me.

Though I always had the best of intentions, always putting patient care first, I reflected on how careless I may have been in taking care of other people while neglecting myself. I knew I could have hurt my family and anyone else with whom I'd been in close proximity. I chided myself for my carelessness, like Superman taking on the cause, thinking I was invincible. Actually, to tell you the truth, I didn't think at all. I just *did*. I've always been a doer, but in the face of a pandemic more is required of me—of each of us—in the realm of how we do things. In that chair by the window I thought a lot about my mother and her lung cancer. My mother died at sixty-five. I was sixty-eight and in many ways believed my life was just beginning. I wanted to do more good! Laguna and the urgent care centers I was going to open were intended to provide my underserved community and others with access to healthcare and a source of income. This would be achieved through operating urgent care and research centers and people's participation in clinical trials. In addition, I hope these efforts will drive more recognition for the region which could serve to bring in more money and more opportunity. What would happen now? I've said it before: I do not want to leave this earth without leaving something behind.

I once heard the Reverend T.D. Jakes say, "Pain always leaves a gift." Clearly it's not always obvious so you have to look for it, and sometimes it's impossibly hard to find. What came of this experience for me were many gifts. In our society we exchange money, but we don't exchange what's really important. Showing and telling people you love them is important. Though the coronavirus put unfathomable constraints on us, God doesn't want us to be alone and certainly not to die alone. He wants us to be part of a family, be it biological or one we create when that's not possible. We are creatures of unity and communication, emotion and interaction. COVID has made so much alien to human nature, to human behavior, resulting in widespread depression and that's not just a byproduct seen in victims of the virus. Granted it has left some with fatigue, brain fog, and low feelings, but depression impacts so many others of us because of what we've gone through mentally and emotionally in just trying to get through the pandemic. Though we have no choice if we want to get to the other side, it's really not okay to be alone. We share pizza and we go out together to movies. We have cookouts together, take vacations, share classrooms, and workplaces. When we're sick, we rely on others to bring us soup, spend time visiting, and sometimes hold us. When it's gone, we're set adrift.

I came back a different person from COVID. It may sound hokey but for the first time I saw life not as something to just power through but to be truly lived My conviction to achieve all I can on this earth was strongly reinforced. But it was also underscored with a marked gratitude for the people making everything in my life possible—especially my family.

I don't typically take naps but in the weeks after I returned home from San Antonio it was a necessity. My recovery was slow and daunting. Rita and Mariellen would force me outside to take steps with the dog and sit in the sun, and even that was exhausting. I lost twenty-two pounds and it took months for my appetite to return. During one of these naps, I dreamed of Dr. Joaquin Cigarroa Jr., a leading physician and probably the most influential physician in Laredo history. His 2019 obituary identified him as the first Harvard Medical School-educated doctor from the Texas-Mexico border. I met with Dr. Cigarroa when I first returned to the area and was setting up my practice. I had received his blessing and my practice thrived.

In the dream he was smiling, communicating not with words but through mental telepathy—which someone later explained to me is the way we are believed to communicate in the afterlife. Dr. Cigarroa "said" he'd touched the face of God and that I should not be afraid. Then I woke up. While I interpreted this as his calling me home, so to speak, most people who've heard this inconceivable story feel it was quite the opposite: while he's telling me there's nothing to fear beyond this life, at the same time I should not be afraid to live out my days. In other words don't waste time thinking about death; just keep living.

I think we all reach out to grab onto something that feeds us and fuels our cause. When I was growing up Laredo had one TV station: KGNS-TV. Today TV goes on twenty-four hours a day, but for those old enough to remember there was the standard sign-off at midnight with the test pattern that looked like an old vinyl 45, followed by static. Often a TV station played the National Anthem. In the case of KGNS-TV, it was the song "You'll Never Walk Alone." My first memory of sitting there listening to it was at the age of two (thank you, mom and dad, for the late night treat), and I never forgot the words. The song is about hope—the courage to walk through a storm and if we can push ourselves do that, to persevere, the good things that await us at the end. My apologies if all this sounds a little saccharine but if you haven't tried it, I strongly prescribe it.

9

In a Post-COVID World

"All that you can take with you is what you've given away." – Anonymous

In the final chapter, I will try and answer the difficult question of where we go from here. If I can inspire you to make changes in the process, I've done what I set out to do. If not, I ask that you simply consider my ideas, taking from them whatever you can use.

How do we navigate a post-COVID world where, in many ways, the term post-COVID is a misnomer? It's possible the virus may not entirely leave us, and in fact I'm convinced it won't. To that end, and for the immediate future, I need to take this final opportunity to implore you to avail yourself of the vaccine. As I said in the beginning, clearly there are elements of our existence we cannot control. I believe it's up to us, even our responsibility, to embrace the ones we can.

We've talked about and I have seen firsthand the long haulers who get the coronavirus and continue to suffer symptoms after they are pronounced healthy again. We've also talked about the virus's repercussions in the form of comorbidities that may show up months and years after the patient appears to have recovered. I've said before, I tend to be an optimist, but nevertheless, who knows? The reality is I may be among them; time will tell.

In what we consider a real accomplishment, Laguna Clinical Research Associates was recently approached to participate in pediatric COVID-19 vaccine studies and is looking forward to the day when children will also be approved to safely receive the vaccine. People ask repeatedly when things will get back to normal and while I believe there will be some return to previous ways of doing things, nothing will be exactly the same. The government will need to adapt and change radically—including economically—to accommodate the fallout, the likes of which we'll not have seen before. That's a lot of negativity from a confessed optimist, but perhaps for the sake of accuracy I can reclassify myself as a kind of hybrid optimist/realist: a "realoptimist." In these unprecedented times, there's really no other way to be. I do, however, believe there is a kind of blueprint we can use for living—something, perhaps unwittingly, I began to think about when I was very sick and very alone, staring out the window for days on end in the San Antonio ICU. So what is it?

Erastus (from the Latin and Greek, meaning "beloved")

How many times have we heard the expression "no guarantees"? At the risk of stating the obvious, we live in an increasingly uncertain world. While my childhood was not perfect, like many of us sometimes I want to catapult myself back, Michael J. Fox-style, and just be there. I still live in Laredo, an amazing community, but like everything else it has grown. With growth, while some things are gained, some are lost.

Ideally I'd like to live in a small town environment much like my own in the 1950s and '60s. If I can share my deepest thoughts with you now, I want my mother to wake me again at dawn on summer days, something she took great care to do before the searing South Texas sun had a chance to bore a hole in my head as I hightailed it out to our jerry-rigged ballfield. My only goal was to share the day with my friends. That's the feeling I'm after: that sense of love, my mother's concern, community, and camaraderie. The way we all supported each other.

I'd like to go back in time to that day in the Concourse Plaza Hotel lobby in Brooklyn, my backside plastered to the couch as I eagerly anticipated a single glimpse, any glimpse, of the New York Yankees who lived there. When Al Downing gave me his autograph, and acknowledged me the next day in the elevator with nice words about me to my mother, that's the kindness I'm after.

When Charlie and I were small, for twenty cents we'd take the bus to the movies. My mother would tell the driver to look out for us which he always did. She also asked the man who owned the movie theatre to keep an eye on us, which he'd do by shining a flashlight on us something like every five minutes (maybe it was ten) to make sure we were okay—and behaving, I'm sure! That man and his wife became patients of mine later in life. Granted, while you could ask people to do things like that more than a half century ago, the world has changed, but it's the thought, the feeling, and the values that I miss. Am I dreaming when I ask if they're all that difficult to replicate in this world? Though they may manifest in a different form, I'm not so sure they are.

I especially wish I could be transported back to a particular day in my small community, emblazoned in my brain, when my little brother and I walked to school, our dog Erastus following close behind. It was long before the days of mandatory leash laws when dogs ran free in the neighborhood, their only responsibility to come home in time for dinner. In Erastus's case, he also assumed the responsibility of walking us, apparently safely, to school. On this day, Charlie stepped off the curb to cross the street. A car came out of nowhere and Erastus grabbed Charlie's pants leg in his teeth, causing him to stop, the dog's courageous, selfless act saving his life. Erastus could have been killed too but his instincts overrode that. Say what you will about animals' ability to reason, but there is no question he put my brother's life first.

So what does that say about us, as human beings, a species that in the face of fear or danger doesn't consider others as much as we could? I'd like to think some of us do, and the following examples are going to demonstrate this, though again it's not always the case. So here's the blueprint for living I mentioned earlier: I firmly believe in order to survive now and in the years to come, we're going to have to do a lot more to take care of other people. My thinking, quite succinctly, is *to make a small town of a big world*, a place defined by compassion, selflessness, altruism, inclusion, encouragement, and overall small town values. All this instead of practicing division, prejudice, fear, anger, and mistrust. The coronavirus with all of its politicizing and polarizing, and its medically necessary separation parameters, has created a microcosm of this country where we've become increasingly isolated from one another. The fact is, though, division, doubt, and apathy are something that started chipping away at our society long before the pandemic, which only seems to have exacerbated it. Perhaps it's time to reconsider the way we live.

When the virus started, Veronica and I went before the staff of our urgent care center. These are frontline workers but we expressed our understanding that if they wanted to opt out of coming to work, we'd support their decision. Not a single one left, saying this is what they signed up for when they went into clinical practice.

Edward Lightner, an R.N. who works long hours for a home health care agency here in Laredo and spends time caring for the elderly in nursing homes as well, regularly showed up at our urgent care center throughout COVID-19. He'd request swabs and I'd ask, sometimes loudly, *"What are you doing here?"* He always said he was going to help me swab my patients, and that was the end of it. No discussion. These people weren't on his home health care agenda and as many times as I tried to pay him for all this extra work, he'd refuse. Many of our frontline workers who elected to keep coming to work did end up with COVID, making Edward's record of showing up that much more heroic. Edward is the kind of human being where if I needed to call him for something at 2 a.m., he'd do it. When we had cars lined up in parking lots, he'd come and help us direct traffic, and swab, coming again and again and again. *That's what he could do.*

Claudia Hourigan, an R.N. and home health agency owner who recently became a nurse practitioner, would regularly show up at my urgent care swab clinic in the summer of 2020 knowing Veronica needed help at the height of all the testing. It wasn't unusual for Veronica to swab fifty, seventy-five, even regularly more than one hundred patients a day, with one medical assistant helping her check IDs and assist patients with consent forms. Claudia was busy, she had a home health agency to run, yet she knew we needed help and realized her patients needed to be protected by increased testing sites in Laredo. *That's what she could do.*

To Serve and Protect

At the beginning of the pandemic, in many venues around the country including ours there was a shortage of surgical and N95 masks.

Sturdily designed, N95 masks are mandated for healthcare workers. Medical personnel were going so far as to put out personal pleas on social media to other medical personnel all over the country to send any available extra masks so they could go in to work. It was a dire situation.

One day a box of masks showed up at the clinic. They were N95s but older models, apparently having sat in a warehouse somewhere. The CDC said it was okay to use old N95 masks as long as there is no other supply and administrative protections (face shields) are in place. We had no choice but to use those masks. The filter was still good but the straps had degraded. A seamstress in our community known by one of our urgent care workers decided she needed to do something, volunteering to make reinforced straps for each and every mask so our healthcare workers could be as protected as possible. That's what I'm talking about, what happens when people think about others. She could have simply sat back, watched TV, and lamented the state of the world. In addition to her job for which I'm sure she put in long hours, she didn't have to spend nights and weekends doing what she did to support Laredo's frontline workers. She took action, figuring out a way to put her skills to work. *That's what she could do.*

Today Asians in this country join the unfortunate ranks of other minority victims in the realm of hate crimes—heinous acts that continue to defy description. Had a virologist in China, a nation supremely blamed for the coronavirus, not taken it upon himself to send the genome to a California research facility in January 2020, we'd not have a vaccine at all. By virtue of this single act, the Asian scientist has now saved millions upon millions of lives all over the world. *That's what he could do.*

Lest We Forget

Sound familiar? The phrase "lest we forget" is commonly used in commemorative and remembrance services, particularly in reference to wartime. Before it was used that way, it was seen eight times in the 1897 Rudyard Kipling poem "Recessional." The actual genesis of the phrase is from a Bible verse in Deuteronomy 4:7-9 and goes like this:

> *For what nation is there so great, who hath God so nigh unto them, as the Lord our God is in all things that we call upon him for? And what nation is there so great, that hath statutes and judgments so righteous as all this law, which I set before you this day?*

> *Only take heed to thyself, and keep thy soul diligently,* **lest thou forget** the things which thine eyes have seen, and *lest they depart* from thy heart all the days of thy life: but teach them thy sons, and thy son›s sons …."

Why am I telling you this? I speak for myself and I think for others when I say it is human nature to get so caught up in the daily struggle we do forget. And when we forget, we repeat the behaviors we shouldn't—behaviors that cause much damage. We forget that not so long ago, Jews and others in Germany, Austria, and Poland were persecuted and slaughtered by the Holocaust. Somehow, thanks to my grandfather, my mother's family got out but I'm certain others in my family perished.

We forget that in WWII Japanese-Americans in this country were forced into internment camps to "prove their loyalty."

In so many ways the nation forgets, but it's important not to. When we find ourselves more inclined to judge, profile, look the other away, dismiss, or just begin to think negatively about others, remembering can make a difference.

In Dreams We Trust

I know I risk being called a dreamer, but what if we all did that? What if we remembered, dreamed, and acted accordingly? The world has been changed by the courage and vision of far more notable dreamers than I, people like Nelson Mandela, John F. Kennedy, Albert Einstein, Thomas Edison, Benjamin Franklin, Mahatma Gandhi, Marie Curie, Martin Luther King Jr., Rosa Parks, and Steve Jobs to name just a few. These are true visionaries— fearless dreamers. The definition of visionary is someone who thinks about the future in a creative or imaginative way. Further defined, a visionary is ahead of his or her time, having a significant concept for change. If the individuals I just mentioned and others never dreamed, never envisioned, nothing in this world would have ever changed.

What about us? Why can't we do that? What's stopping us? There are people out there without Nobel Peace Prizes, football-sized factories, or entire laboratories or countries behind them, yet they've taken small steps toward transforming classrooms or neighborhoods, even helping just one neighbor at a time, changing the way we think and what's possible as a result. Though it may be easier said than done (most things don't come easy, right?), I offer up my *make a small town of a big world* blueprint as a call to action.

When I was growing up, we knew the Ramirez family next door and the Chapmans across the street. We knew when Mrs. Ramirez was nursing a badly burned finger and ran out of tortillas, so we brought her some. In Laredo we made it a point to know and help our neighbors, no matter what their religion, ethnicity, political beliefs, or something they may have said to us one day in anger, frustration, fear, or sadness.

In the early 1970s, one of my mother's best friends passed away. My mother went to the funeral and then back to the family's house to sit Shiva—a Jewish tradition where family and friends come together to pray, share food, and reminisce about the deceased. My mother walked up to the sister of the departed to express her condolences, a level of grief my mother felt deeply within herself as well having lost a very close friend, whereby the sister told her it should have been my mother who died instead. While clearly a shocking, hurtful scenario, my mother rose above it, embracing this woman anyway, knowing sometimes we're so consumed by our circumstances we need grace and understanding to begin healing. I never forgot the story, the way Rosa Haber acted in the face of suffering and personal attack, opening her heart to this woman nevertheless in the woman's darkest hour.

I wish to thank you for the privilege of your time in reading this book. Your interest in learning something of my life, and considering the dreams I have for myself and for each of us, is your gift to me. The gift I have to offer in return is in the form of a question, perhaps a challenge. At this point, knowing what you do now, how will you choose to live in a post-COVID world?

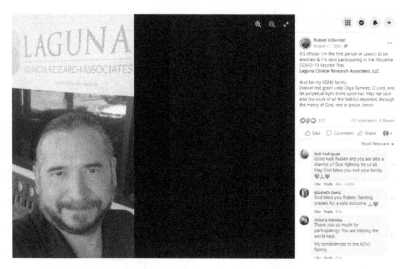

Ruben Villarreal, KGNS News, the very first person to be
vaccinated in Laredo, TX through the Moderna study

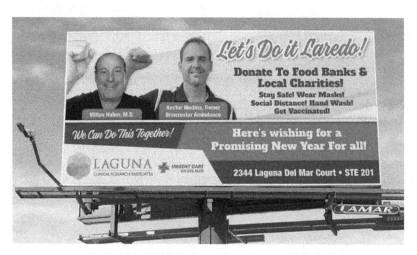

Hector Medina, Owner of BronzeStar Ambulance, (right) with
me on a local Laredo billboard encouraging our community
during the height of the pandemic (December 2020)

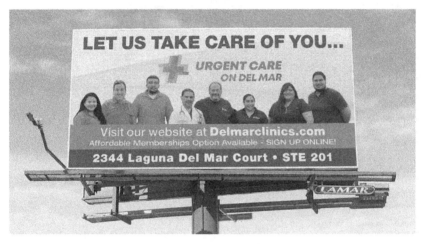

My urgent care staff (to the left) and me (center) with my research staff (to the right) all vaccinated by their own choices, as we transition into a Post-Pandemic mindset (June 2021)

Acknowledgments

Thank you to all frontline workers everywhere who fought and continue to fight the COVID pandemic. You are truly the heroes.

To all my Nurse Practitioners, including Ron Meza, Marco Vela, and Steve Zurita, my staff, and clinical workers, including Cesar Flores. You stuck by my side during the uncertainty of the pandemic, risking your lives to provide our services to the community. May you continue to do great things.

To Robert Schnitzler, M.D. and all my other treating physicians for being there to encourage me and help me through my Covid battle. I appreciate your dedication and am honored to be among you.

To all the patients, their families, and other loved ones who lost their lives to COVID. May you find comfort in knowing the vaccine will prevent a future like the past.

My deepest appreciation to the clinical trial participants in in South Texas, the United States, and the entire world. You bravely volunteered and continue to participate in the quest to eradicate the coronavirus. Without you, we would lose the battle.

My inexpressible gratitude to the residents of my hometown of Laredo, Texas. You helped bring new medicine and new horizons to our community by participating in and endorsing ongoing clinical research. I am proud to live here among you.

To Rita, Paul, and Mariellen Haber. You lifted me up when I fell down, physically and spiritually. You are the backbone of my life and I am forever grateful.

To my extended family and all my colleagues and friends, thank-you.

To my compadres and travel companions Hector Medina and Joe Sillas for your unwavering friendship and support throughout all phases of my life. Thank-you for being by my side and, Hector Medina, for driving me to San Antonio in your ambulance when I had Covid. Both of your lives have made mine richer.

My sincere appreciation to Victor Trevino, M.D., Health Authority for the city of Laredo, for your tireless dedication in leading our city through the pandemic and serving as an invaluable resource to our community overall.

My great thanks to U.S. Congressman Henry Cuellar, 28th Congressional District, for your contributions in furthering crucial clinical research in South Texas.

About the Author

Milton Haber, M.D., grew up the baseball-obsessed son of a driven Laredo, Texas business owner from whom he got his work ethic. His mother, who fled Poland for Mexico as a child, taught him compassion, a catalyst for his career in internal medicine. Boyhood trips to Mexican relatives exposed him to the indescribable poverty and suffering of strangers along the way, further directing the course of his life. He routinely provided food, medicine, rent money, and more to his patients in need.

In 2018, at an age when many retire, he expanded the scope of his mission. Founding Laguna Clinical Research Associates to facilitate life-changing clinical trials in his Laredo community and eventually throughout South Texas, studies would include Moderna's COVID-19 vaccine trials. Contracting the coronavirus himself, a life and death ICU experience set him on a spiritual path where he created a blueprint for navigating a post-COVID world.

Beth Herman is a journalist, author, editor, and Amazon #1 bestselling ghostwriter of more than 20 books ranging from business and finance to architecture and design, lifestyle and healthy living, religion and spirituality, memoir and business memoir, and animal welfare. Her features and profiles have appeared in the Washington Post, Cape Cod Times, Portland Press Herald, Los Angeles Times Syndicate, Farmers' Almanac, Harvard Divinity School Annual Report and more. She received her Bachelor of Arts from Brandeis University and lives in coastal Maine.

CPSIA information can be obtained
at www.ICGtesting.com
Printed in the USA
LVHW050538130721
692517LV00001B/72